Thyroid & Menopause Madness

Why It Feels Like You're Falling Apart and What You Can Do About It

BY JONI LABBE,
DC, CCN, DCCN

Published by Blue Ground Publishing

First Edition: 2015 as "Why Is Mid-Life Mooching Your Mojo?"

ISBN: 978-1-7031416-2-7 (paperback)

ISBN: 978-0-9971797-4-3 (ebook)

Library of Congress Control Number: 2014921907

Joni's 21st century book, written in a highly readable, useful, and practical style, shows women how they can continue to have a full, passionate, and energetic life. Dr. Labbe shows how the typical problems women experience in their mid-life can be not only managed, but overcome.

— Richard W. Levak, Ph.D. Consultant to reality TV programs such as Survivor, Big Brother, Amazing Race, and the Apprentice

If you suffer with an autoimmune disease, or have a stressed out life, you will love this book. You will love Dr. Labbe, and she will get to the root problem. She has helped many of my patients overcome insomnia, digestive issues, hot flashes, and brain fog, and has my highest respect for the way she explains complicated material in an easy, fun, understandable format.

— Al A. Fallah, DDS, FICCMO, AIAOMT

Over the last ten years of transitioning from conventional allopathic medicine to the present functional medicine model, I have seen that the chiropractors and other alternative practitioners are leading the way to a new, natural approach to healing, and Dr. Labbe is in the forefront of this movement. Her book provides the full perspective of healing in a concise, easy to read format, and references to get additional help, if needed.

— Juergen Winkler, MD Quantum Functional Medicine

This book offers straightforward strategies for understanding and improving health in mid-life in a compelling, light-hearted, easy to follow format. Let Dr. Labbe guide you on the path to discovering your missing mojo; it worked for me and it will work for you.

— Kathryn Rudlin, LCSW Author of: Ghost Mothers: Healing From the Pain of a Mother Who Wasn't Really There

DEDICATION

I want to thank and dedicate this book to the many caring women who have so graciously shared their pain, stories, and healing victories with me. These committed women have not been afraid to change, implement, and go the distance, despite tremendous pain and fatigue, while getting to the root cause of their health issues. You are true heroes; I admire, love and respect you. Each of you has inspired me to finally get my message into book form, in order to share the trials and adventures of how to regain hope, vitality, and passion.

I also offer my gratitude and appreciation to Dr. Datis Kharrazian, for his revolutionary healing protocols for Hashimoto's disease and hypothyroidism. My deepest thanks for his tireless work that has enabled me to better serve and enhance the lives of my clients.

Most importantly, I dedicate this book to my husband Jim, who has provided tremendous support, advice, and assistance. Without his patience, love, and inspiration while I was writing this book, this would not have been possible.

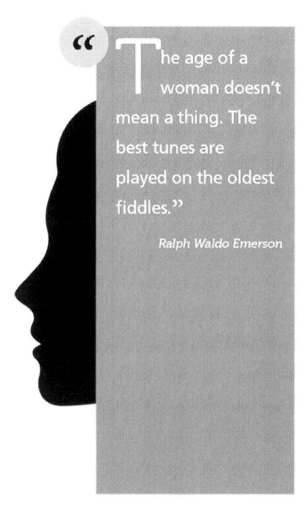

"The age of a woman doesn't mean a thing. The best tunes are played on the oldest fiddles."

Ralph Waldo Emerson

Table of Contents

FOREWORD

Here's the bad news about living in our modern world: staying well as we age can be complicated. Even with the best of intentions, life—with all its inherent stresses—takes over and "me-time" essentially disappears as children, job and significant others get top billing. Before you know it, entropy sets in and we begin feeling our age. In the blink of an eye, we are at the midway point and beyond. Unless you lead a charmed life, your mind, body and spirit have taken a bit of a beating. As Dr. Joni says so well, midlife begins "mooching your mojo!"

Here's the good news: there's hope! The human mind, body and spirit are remarkably resilient and there is a way back to health for you. Science has come a long way in understanding the many ways in which our physical health and emotional well-being begin to suffer as we age. When you truly understand these underlying causes, you can begin to correct them one at a time and the healing process begins. More importantly, so does your joy of living.

These foundational principles for healing come from the game-changing new medical field called functional medicine, where we treat causes and not symptoms. Because every one of us is biochemically and genetically unique, these differences must be taken into account or you will become just another victim of the broken medical system that tries to pound a square peg into a round hole by prescribing medications that cover up symptoms instead of treating the underlying causes.

Fortunately for you, Dr. Joni Labbe does a remarkable job of translating these powerful principles into a clear and individualized path that you can start today to begin reclaiming your physical health and emotional well-being. And she does so in a delightful and entertaining way that makes it truly fun to learn and grow and get well again.

Even more importantly, Dr. Labbe's concise, caring and compassionate approach comes not only from an academic interest in the subject, but also from her own personal struggle with autoimmune disease. She has been where you are, felt what you feel and knows the joy you will experience when you too become well again. Dr. Labbe is a remarkable healer and in the true sense of the word, she wants you to become whole again. As you explore these powerful healing principles and apply them to your life, you will feel her concern, her passion and her heartfelt desire to truly help you feel well again. I cannot think of a better guide to take you on this journey of healing than Dr. Labbe. Enjoy your way back to health and vitality.

Neil F. Neimark, M.D.
Body/Soul Connection Newsletters

PREFACE

I am sure you have been seeing a number of books on women's health addressing topics from hormone replacement to diet and life style, but are you seeing books that address all these topics as they relate to one another? Most are only dealing with part of the problem. If you are currently experiencing poor health you should be asking yourself: Am I having an autoimmune problem? Have I been over stressing my adrenal glands? Am I eating too much sugar? Why am I feeling so tired? If you are seeking the full perspective in healing, this book provides answers in a concise, easy to read format and includes references to get additional help, if needed.

All too often in our practice we are seeing the depression of midlife, the weight gain, and the hormonal imbalances. With 20 years in family practice I can attest to this and that the present orthodox approach that prescribes anti-depressants, cholesterol medication, and synthetic hormones to "make one feel better" clearly are not working. In our society we are seeing a growing dissatisfaction with doctors addressing symptoms and not the underlying causes; and there is a shift in the medical care model to better address the root cause of the health problems women are suffering from. The Internet has made this information much more accessible and the timing for Dr. Labbe's book could not be better.

The health problems of today are multi-factorial and Dr. Joni Labbe is giving you a concise approach to unravel the complex problems that are not solved with medication. Each aspect of common health problems for women are addressed individually and then tied back together into a life style approach you can live with. Her approach makes sense, the evidence supports it, and the results are certain to get your health and life back on track.

There is so much information packed into the following pages, so hold onto your hat and don't hesitate to get started. It may feel like you are sacrificing much in the beginning, but once you begin seeing the benefits for yourself and your family, the changes are self-perpetuating. Get ready to make a new life for yourself and begin feeling the zest for life those before you are already enjoying.

Juergen Winkler, MD
Quantum Functional Medicine, Carlsbad, CA

INTRODUCTION
WHY IS MID-LIFE MOOCHING YOUR MOJO?

"Vaginal atrophy," she snorted with indignation. "What god-awful thing is that?"

I was sitting across the desk from a 53-year-old postmenopausal woman. She was in my office seeking help for fatigue, low libido, hair loss, weight gain, and insomnia. Lauren had been to many doctors looking for ways to cope with these issues.

"I'm not done living!" Lauren despaired. "Why do so many doctors keep making me feel like a loser?"

Like a lot of us who live into our 40s and 50s and beyond, Lauren was not lazy, crazy, or finished. But doctors had made her feel that way. Just because every woman goes through menopause does not lessen the devastating impact it can have on our health and lives. Few women talk about it, and if they do, it's often the butt of a joke or casually dismissed.

Transitioning into menopause can be a nasty slap in the face for many of us. Here we are buzzing along through life. The kids are finally at an age where we can complete a thought. We're hitting our stride in our career, perhaps at last earning a respectable income and professional respect.

And then what happens? Bam! Suddenly the periods come every two weeks in torrential gushes, or whenever they please. **Hot flashes threaten to ignite our thinning hair, and now we need to shave our faces?** Just when we're commanding respect at work, a mysterious fog shrouds our brains, slowing function to a crawl. Memory is contained on Post-it Notes and iPhone calendar alerts. Strange 'demons' periodically possess us, and we yell, cry, or both for no particular reason. Sex hurts, but who wants to do that anymore anyway? It's like the Sahara Desert down there. And sleep. Oh, we long for precious sleep, but here we are wide-awake in the wee hours of the morning, night after night. Sneeze, laugh, or chug some water and we're wetting our underwear. New layers of fat turn up in the oddest places (back fat, really?), taking the fun out of wearing clothes. Weird things start popping up at checkups, like high blood pressure. To add insult to injury, the hair salon recommends a product for aging hair, and the eye doctor says it's time for bifocals.

And here's the thing – we cope, we manage, we smile, we pretend we are OK. We pick up the pieces of our health and carry on. We look perfectly normal while shopping at the grocery store, and yet it seems like our body is slowly disintegrating, slowly developing strange new symptoms. How concerned do we need to be? Will anything help? Doctors tend to dismiss our complaints with prescriptions for antidepressants, anti-anxiety meds, and sleeping pills. These solutions rarely help. But we know; deep down we know this is not who we are, this is not how it's supposed to be. This is NOT OK!

If men went through menopause, a national emergency would have been declared long ago! Hundreds of millions of dollars poured into research, and the topic would be headline news. Every hospital would have a menopause wing; millions would bravely participate in menopause fun runs and proudly wear little menopause ribbons, blood-red maybe. Retired football players would do menopause ads on TV. We'd talk about it with a serious tone at

Starbucks. But no, as women we are too often dismissed, ignored, or even ridiculed. Sometimes our husbands divorce us, or doctors send us on our way with an ever expanding list of prescriptions.

I'm painting a pretty dire picture, even though I left out a lot of symptoms. I know that a woman can suffer from extreme menopausal symptoms and still patch together a pretty decent life. Plenty do, because women are incredibly strong by the time we hit midlife. It's kind of like labor and birth. Only this time the pain and discomfort are drawn out over many years. Older women in our lives pat us on the back with a compassionate smile and assure us we will get through this. **Things will get better, we're told, but they never really do for a lot of women.**

Here's the thing, although menopause is perfectly normal, suffering grievously through this transition and losing your health is not. Not for Lauren, not for me, and not for you. This is largely a modern malady. When the ovaries wind down and eventually stop making estrogen, the adrenal glands are designed to pick up the slack and produce the hormones we need to function normally. The problem is that by the time Lauren and many other American women hit their 40s, their adrenal glands (two glands that sit atop the kidneys and look like walnuts), are now like two little burnt pieces of toast. Why? The adrenal glands manage stress, and the poor things have been worked to the bone. By midlife they are tuckered out, barely managing their most basic functions, much less able to take on something as significant as estrogen production. So estrogen gets moved to the bottom of the to-do list, the ovaries have a going-out-of-business sale, and the many estrogen dependent tissues in your body, particularly your brain, are left gasping at a dry well.

It doesn't have to be this way. My friend Lisa says menopause is when the 'chickens come home to roost.' All the transgressions of youth come back to haunt you during the transition into menopause. You can no longer get away with never sleeping, eating like a teenager, and thinking exercise is only for the spunky spandex girls at the gym. It's time now to do the work that's needed to take care of your body.

After my visit with Lauren, I thought back to my own midlife journey. I had been enjoying a long, rewarding career as a chiropractor specializing in nutrition. I had earned my degree as a Board Certified Clinical Nutritionist. I even hosted a two-hour talk radio show, "Healthier Way with Dr. Labbe" on a San Diego radio station, and enjoyed my community of family and friends. But there were small insidious changes that I chalked up to age, or menopause, or life. I had a hard time taking 10 lbs off even though I worked out (before going into the office) and ate "right." I had a little brain fog: *why did I walk into the room, where did I park the car?* Sleep was restless, and I kept waking up at 3:00 am. It was time to get real with myself. I had put on extra stubborn weight and felt "foggy-brained" ever since going through menopause. My memory wasn't as sharp as it used to be, and I got tired more easily. I thought it was just age, or that I was doing too much.

As I do with all my clients, I run blood work on myself every year. In 2007, in my early 50s, the blood report showed the presence of antibodies. In that moment, I felt my stomach drop to my knees. I knew exactly what this meant; it was a result I had seen often on the blood work reports of my patients. You could have bowled me over with a feather! I was in the health and wellness world. I walked the talk! I took supplements, exercised, managed my stress, and practiced my faith.

How could I have been doing everything right and have a test result like this? I had developed an autoimmune hypothyroidism condition called Hashimoto's disease. This is an autoimmune disease in which the thyroid gland is attacked by a variety of cell and antibody-mediated immune processes. Hashimoto's often results in hypothyroidism with bouts of hyperthyroidism. But that was only part of the puzzle! I also learned, through additional testing, that I have Celiac disease, an autoimmune intolerance to gluten.

After I picked myself off the floor and licked my wounds, I went on a quest to find out how I could "live big" with two autoimmune diseases. I read books by Mary Shoman, a magnificent patient advocate and prolific writer on thyroid and autoimmune issues. It was an honor to study with the brilliant Dr. Datis Kharrizan, and I leaned in to learn all I could: for my own quality of life and to empower others with what worked (and what didn't).

This is how my journey started, desperate for answers for my own survival and curious about all the pieces of the puzzle. How could I get to the root cause of the problem, and how could I implement meaningful changes in practical ways? Over time the process that you will learn from this book emerged. **It's the process of identifying all the pieces of your health puzzle** and then putting them together in a way that enables a healthy, vibrant you. This process has brought energy back to my life, and to the lives of the clients I've had the privilege to serve.

Scared into Action

That blood test scared me into action. As a clinician I know about autoimmune disease and have seen what it does to people. One autoimmune disease often leads to another, and then another. If Hashimoto's disease is left untreated, you can eventually find yourself dealing with pernicious anemia, type 1 diabetes, or multiple sclerosis; all very real possibilities that I've learned about first-hand in my practice. I immediately went on a strict gluten-free diet because of what I had learned studying with Dr. Datis Kharrazian, DHSc, DC, MS; author of *Why Do I Still Have Thyroid Symptoms?* and *Why Isn't My Brain Working?* I also applied what I learned from Dr. Bob Marshall, founder of Premiere Labs and Quantum Reflex Analysis, and Sam Queen, research director of The Institute for Health Realities. I consolidated all this knowledge to put together a supplement and diet regimen for myself based on my lab tests and symptoms. I was on a mission to get back the mojo that my menopause had mooched. This has been my passion and what I have specialized in since my diagnosis in 2007.

It can be difficult to achieve vibrant health, and it takes time. Discovering I had Hashimoto's was just the first piece of the puzzle. I also discovered that Celiac disease, hormonal imbalances, gut health, and numerous other factors contributed to my symptoms. It took some time to find all the pieces, but once I did I had an overall picture of what my body needed for optimum health. Then, all that was left was to commit to doing whatever it took to achieve it.

The first 30 days required some real discipline, but I lost 10 pounds in the first six weeks and my brain fog lifted. I developed a greater sense of well-being, and was sleeping better, and waking refreshed. This was quite motivating and made it easier to stick to the diet and the protocol. However, midlife offers no free passes—we spent all those in our youth. Every day I have to pay attention to my diet, engage in physical activity, manage stress, and take a few key supplements (not a whole kitchen counter full). I will need to keep this up for the rest of my life, because I've learned this is what my body requires to maintain vibrant health. There is no "cure" for Hashimoto's/low thyroid, no "magic bullet," but in this book you'll learn how to successfully piece together your own health, easily manage your condition, get your life back, and live big until God calls you home.

I exercise four to five times a week, pray every morning for wisdom and every night for forgiveness. Gluten and junk foods no longer tempt me, and I now enjoy excellent health, balanced thyroid function, and an inspiring midlife – no longer fretting about low energy, brain fog, or weight gain.

Join me on this journey, this exciting and empowering adventure. I will share with you, as I have with hundreds of other women, health guidance that works so you can have your life, your brain, and your sexuality back, and maybe lose some of the back fat! You can enjoy your body again instead of feeling imprisoned by it, and you can **get back to the glorious business of being fully alive, instead of just getting through the day.**

Growing up With an Unwell Mom

I lost my mom to breast cancer when she was only 50; I was 20 years old when she died. I know firsthand what it's like to lose a loved one too soon. I also know how health issues change the dynamics of the whole family, especially when it is Mom who is unwell. My mom was full of hope, dreams, and life. But as far back as I can remember, my mom was often asleep right after dinner, or too tired to make dinner. She was constantly looking for something that would restore her vitality as she raised her three daughters, tried to maintain friendships, and enjoy my dad and life's little pleasures. She tried so hard to live, but poor health robbed her of that opportunity.

Now when I look back, I believe that my mother suffered from undiagnosed hypothyroidism, insulin resistance, and adrenal fatigue. I also believe that a stressful childhood with an alcoholic father, the loss of her fiancé in World War II, an undiagnosed gluten intolerance, and a mouth full of mercury fillings contributed to her lack of energy, inability to lose weight, brain fog, and early death. I know the particular hardships of being raised by a mother who suffers from chronically poor health. When women who struggle as my mother did come into my office desperate for help, often after having seen multiple doctors, my heart goes out to them, because I grew up with someone just like that.

Nine years after my mother died I lost my dad to melanoma at the age of 60. I had buried both my parents by the time I was 30. These experiences taught me that every minute that goes by can never be won back. I watched my mother suffer for too many years from conditions I now know could have been easily managed. **There is no excuse today; we have the knowledge and tools to stay healthy.** Your local MD might not, but the researchers are all over it, and thanks to mega-minds like Dr. Datis Kharrazian and other functional medicine educators, we are bringing this research to women who are ready to reclaim their mojo.

My Quest to Help Others with Health Challenges

I was compelled to write this book by the many women who come to me who have seen specialists and gotten no answers; who leave doctors' offices feeling resentful because of the implication that they are hypochondriacs, inventing their complaints, seeking attention, or just being a nuisance.

Women are often told, "Take this medication." Or, "You're just getting older." In other words, how dare you expect to live a healthy, fulfilling life you selfish whiner! Now be a good girl and be quiet.

Doctors aren't bad people. I think most go into their profession because they genuinely want to help people, but they are limited by a lack of knowledge. We don't know what we don't know. The tragedy of medicine today is that the science is out there, the researchers are on it, but somehow the information is not trickling down into the office of the ordinary MD, many of whom still practice outdated, pharmaceutical-based medicine.

This leads me to the heart and soul of this book: *What if you knew which tests to run and what problems to target? What if you knew the underlying cause of your multitude of symptoms? What if you could reclaim your health and become the beautiful, mojo-brandishing woman warrior you were meant to be? What if you had all the pieces of the puzzle laid out for you—and had the motivation and support to rebuild your health?* Knowledge is the ultimate power, and that is what I'm here to deliver. It is the mystery, the not knowing, that drives people crazy with despair when they're feeling unwell. When you understand your body, understand where things are breaking down, and the symptoms this breakdown causes, you have the needed tools to do something about it. You have the power. **Your body has the inborn ability to recover, to heal.** You just need to know what steps and actions to take.

It is rare for medical issues to be based on a lack of pharmaceuticals. Make no mistake: I'm not against medication, if you truly need it. Drugs can be lifesaving or help improve comfort, but you should always hunt for the reason *why* you need the meds, and address what is causing your symptoms.

This book is for every woman who has ever felt frustrated or stuck with the solutions of conventional or even alternative medicine. I have successfully used my method of "Testing, Not Guessing" with hundreds of patients. My powerful solutions are for any woman who feels her life is over, or that she has forever lost her mojo because she is going through midlife changes. Using the recommendations in this book will give you back the power that comes from feeling vibrant, sexy, and clearheaded.

I will give you the needed tools to help you reinvent yourself so you can transform from a domesticated house cat into the proud lioness you were designed to be (or a cougar, if you're into that!). Do not succumb to "this is just the way it is," and do not waste time thinking you are not important enough or your needs aren't justified. You need to feel better because the world needs you. It needs each of us, and we need to be able to feel and function better to take our place in the world.

This conviction is what set me on a quest to study "functional medicine," a form of medicine that treats underlying causes and is focused on prevention. This is why I have such a passion for my work and for you. My life's work is about preventing degenerative disease and getting to the root cause of the problem, so that you will live a full, long life. I want you to realize how precious you are to your family and friends, and how your life explodes with blessings. **You are never too old, too young, or too sick to start on the road to recovery.**

Every day I'm blessed to counsel people like you to help them develop extraordinary, life-changing habits for optimal health. When my female clients regain their mojo, they positively influence their family and friends, and more powerfully direct their future. The plans I've designed and lay out in this book have been effective for many women around the country. Failure is not an option when you follow the steps and suggestions described in this book.

A Note on Hormone Replacement Therapy

This is not a book about hormone replacement therapy (HRT), as replacing dwindling female hormones is now called. It is an important subject for many perimenopausal and postmenopausal women, and one that has gotten a bad rap due to misinformation and misunderstanding. I do not work with HRT; instead I help my patients to resolve underlying breakdowns in health that contribute to their symptoms, including hormone deficiencies or excesses.

I am not opposed to HRT. If you suffer from irresolvable estrogen deficiency, you are at risk for numerous health problems in your brain and body, including heart disease, Alzheimer's disease, and osteoporosis. (I suggest reading Outliving Your Ovaries by Marina Johnson for a comprehensive review of the research.) However, I believe this treatment should be a last resort except after surgically induced menopause, and should not be undertaken without also addressing what caused your hormonal deficiencies in the first place. Also, addressing your core health issues will help HRT work better, and at smaller doses.

Please do not take the subject of hormone replacement lightly. Do your due diligence to find a qualified, experienced practitioner. HRT is extremely powerful and can cause serious problems if prescribed improperly. Make sure to use only bioidentical (natural) hormones as opposed to synthetic, topical, or oral estrogen at the most conservative doses possible, and get your hormone levels tested regularly. Symptoms of hormone deficiency and hormone excess can overlap, and the dosage varies from woman to woman. HRT is not without its risks, but the risks of bioidentical hormones are now understood to be much smaller than once believed.

The tools I discuss in this book are vital to minimizing your risk of disease and may even reduce the risks associated with HRT. Your body is a complex machine that needs careful feeding and attention. **Do not take better care of your car or your house than you do your own body.** Make the functioning of your body a top priority and only work with doctors who treat it the same way. You are NOT crazy, lazy, or finished! I know that you can regain your mojo and vibrant health! ThyroSisters, you are not alone. We will do this together!

PART ONE:
Picking Up The Pieces:
Where, Oh Where,
Has My Mojo Gone?

CHAPTER 1

THE FIRST PIECE OF THE PUZZLE:
You're Not Lazy, Crazy or Finished

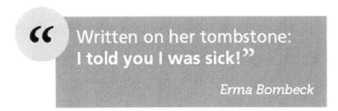

" Written on her tombstone:
I told you I was sick!**"**

Erma Bombeck

Michelle was a well-educated woman in her early 50s, and the mother of two college students. I knew right away that Michelle was a unique and special person, but her story was all too familiar. She was physically falling apart, having been to the Mayo Clinic, acupuncturists, chiropractors, naturopaths, MD's, and faith healers – all to no avail.

One doctor told Michelle she might have fibromyalgia. Others said she suffered from depression and anxiety, and that taking an antidepressant might help. She came to my office looking and feeling weary. Her skin was darkening, her hair thinning. She simply had no gas left in the tank.

"I have a good marriage," Michelle said. "It seems like just yesterday I was full of life and energy. But I am terrified. It was all I could do to drag myself into your office today." Michelle wiped at her big brown eyes. "Doctors can't find anything wrong, and all of my blood work is normal. I really can't point to anything causing my insomnia, depression, and weight gain. Yes, I have stress, but it's not overwhelming. Simple tasks like getting dinner on the table are sometimes too much. The brain fog is unrelenting. I try to form sentences, but the words don't come out." Her hands trembled as she choked out her story. "I can't remember why I walked into a room. I can't remember my friends' names. I'm falling apart."

Michelle reported that whenever she talked about not feeling well her family changed the subject. Her poor health was beginning to strain her marriage. "I love my husband, but I have no libido. Intercourse is painful sometimes, and frankly I'm just not interested. I'm so tired all day, and my joints hurt. I know I'm too young to feel this way, but my friends and doctors chalk it all up to aging."

Michelle's confidence had been shattered by ongoing, unrelenting health problems, and her emotions were stretched to the breaking point. **She felt like she was dying, but all her lab test results came back 'normal**,' suggesting there was nothing medically wrong with her. Therefore, others concluded that she must be lazy, crazy, or finished. But Michelle, like the hundreds of women I talk to and work with across the country, is far from finished with her life. Yet because she could not be diagnosed with a disease or assigned an insurance code, doctors dismissed her complaints, or decided she was suffering from depression or anxiety.

We needed to get to the root of what was causing Michelle's symptoms. By running blood tests to include a comprehensive metabolic panel, a complete thyroid panel (including T3, T4, T7), a CBC with differentials, plus thyroid antibodies (TPO and TBG), (I will share with you what all these tests mean later in the book) we learned that Michelle has Hashimoto's disease, an autoimmune thyroid disease that affects more women than men, and is the most under-diagnosed autoimmune disease in the US. (I will talk about Hashimoto's in more depth later in this book.) The tests revealed that she also has a "leaky gut," which causes chronic inflammation in the body. Michelle followed a protocol I designed for her of science-based nutritional therapy, functional neurological treatments, and a gluten-free, dairy-free diet. Within six weeks the brain fog disappeared, her spirits lifted, and she felt sexual for the first time in years.

The experience for women suffering from undiagnosed midlife symptoms often goes like this in terms of how others respond: How dare you be so self-centered as to talk about your health needs. How dare you value yourself enough to keep trying to feel better. How dare you demand to feel good. In other words: Accept that you are an aging woman of fading beauty who has no energy, a lackluster sex life, and the inability to remember your own children's names.

The saddest thing is how common Michelle's story is. I have heard similar stories from many of my female clients around the country. Their health problems are chronic and insidious; their symptoms perplex doctors and frustrate family members, because these women generally 'look' okay. Hey, you're not in a wheelchair, you're not disfigured or bandaged up, you're not laying mangled on a stretcher, so therefore you must be fine… quit complaining! And yet the reality is you've lost all joy in living, it's a struggle to read an article and recall it two days later, it's difficult to enjoy your children or grandchildren, and many of the dreams you had for the future now seem impossible.

Searching for the Cause of Your Symptoms

As a post-menopausal woman successfully living with both Hashimoto's and celiac disease, I have been where you are now. Additionally, I have had the pleasure of helping many women get back their midlife mojo by working through a scientific process of detection and diagnosis and then implementing specific steps to bring about healing.

In this book I will introduce you to what underlies the chronic midlife symptoms that are sapping your mojo, explain how to uncover your specific issues (because one symptom can have numerous causes), and show you how to reinvent yourself and your life. I hope in this small way I can give back to all the courageous women I have met over the years who persevered to overcome their fears: the fear that no answers existed, that they were going crazy, that the medical system had failed them, and that there was no way to get their lives back on track.

The explanations in this book are different from the approach provided by your managed-care doctor who is not trained to treat chronic and autoimmune issues or female midlife health issues, because these are health problems for which no magic bullet medication or surgery exists.

This book is founded on functional medicine, a science-based form of medicine that looks to correct the underlying causes of symptoms, versus sweeping them under the rug with drugs or surgery. The emphasis with the functional medicine approach is on correcting faulty function through changes in diet and lifestyle and customized supplementation. I use lab testing to identify problems or trends toward disease and follow-up testing to see if the treatment plan is showing success. I use different ranges on blood tests than the standard lab ranges your doctor probably orders, which primarily target only sickness and disease.

The narrower ranges used in functional medicine represent the ranges used in this country for 30 years, before they were broadened so that more people will fall into "normal" and not burden the managed health care system. This is why you are being told "you are normal, you're fine, you just need antidepressants." If this were back in the 1980's in the regular medical model, the Doctor would have looked at the functional or narrower ranges as the standard of care, and addressed them. I look at both ranges with you: the ranges that would have been flagged were we living before the managed care era, and the broader ranges. If your results lie outside the narrower functional medicine ranges, but are still within today's standard ranges, it may indicate you are moving toward disease. While many doctors might not highlight this important fact, taking action to bring these values back into functional medicine ranges could mean preventing certain diseases altogether.

I want to share some ideas from Dr. Scott Theirl, a well-known functional neurologist and lecturer, who graciously agreed to summarize his views on why the functional approach to healing is so successful. He also introduces many of the healing tools embraced and discussed in more depth in this book.

For thirteen years I have practiced a comprehensive approach to the health of the brain and the body, and am continually amazed at the new healthcare options available with each passing year. When we take a look at the big picture, a '10,000-foot view of health', it is clear that the nervous system, endocrine (hormone), and immune systems are continually playing off one another.

The power of any one system to influence the others is a constant reality.

It is only in recent years that providers have had the objective tests needed to evaluate individual patients as true individuals, and we now recognize that patients can have similar complaints of fatigue, pain, brain fog, moodiness and insomnia, but may have different biologic reasons for their complaints. This is truly a time in integrative healthcare when practitioners can offer personalized road maps to optimal health and improved aging.

These health road maps require the collection of biomarkers as a starting point, so you have to be ready to collect saliva, urine, blood, and possibly stool samples. From these samples, specialized laboratories provide great insight into immune system function and inflammatory processes, nervous system function, neurotransmitter stress responses, and endocrine (hormone) system function, to include hormone imbalances. As clinicians, our goal is to discover which system is having the greatest difficulty functioning at this moment in time. Integrated and comprehensive care clinicians recognize that as we support one system, the others also respond, and thus all positive test findings in all three systems must be optimized and monitored to achieve feeling your best.

The question, "How did I get to this place of feeling so bad?" is often asked of me, and the reality is that there are many reasons that humans become metabolically fatigued. The typical diet is one of pro-inflammatory foods that cause major shifts in blood sugar and are stressful to the immune system. The immune system also has a toxic load to balance that is continually increasing with new synthetic chemicals and more electromagnetic pollution. Some of these chemicals are hormone disruptors and can challenge the natural balance of our sex and thyroid hormones. Living hard and fast most of the time with poor quality sleep is a 21st century challenge. It is impossible to go "full throttle" all day without replenishing ourselves at night with quality, restful sleep.

Chronic stress, whether physical (pain), emotional or cognitive places strain on our neurotransmitters and stress hormones, and leads to imbalances in stress hormones, thyroid hormones, sex hormones and neurotransmitters. Which system fatigues first in any given patient can only be determined by a thorough history, and confirmed with laboratory testing. We are all individuals, each different genetically, and we fatigue our brain and body systems at different rates. This is both the challenge and the opportunity in an integrative healthcare approach.

In summary, start with a great night's sleep, eat well and as organic a diet as possible, engage in physical activity daily, minimize stress of all types, take breaks from technology, think positive, laugh often, love fully, test and optimize your nervous, endocrine and immune systems and enjoy living and aging as it was meant to be...a very good thing.

In identifying the root causes of the symptoms you're experiencing, there are a number of 'usual suspects' to consider, imbalances and issues that can throw your body seriously out of whack. These are introduced below and will be discussed in more depth in the chapters to follow.

THE OVERLOOKED SUSPECTS

1. Poor diet or undiagnosed food allergies
2. Impaired thyroid functioning
3. Compromised immune system
4. Blood sugar imbalances
5. Adrenal fatigue
6. Brain impairment
7. The negative impact of environmental toxins

Is Your Diet Sabotaging Your Health?

Food is either your medicine or your poison. Unfortunately, the food industry in this country is built around poisoning us slowly and sweetly. Foods that are quick, easy, starchy, and sweet underpin the epidemics of obesity, diabetes, dementia, heart disease, and pretty much every chronic disease that is slowly destroying the health of this nation.

Your most powerful therapy, and often the easiest way to get your mojo back, is to improve your diet. Sure, you can get away with eating whatever junk you want in your 20s and 30s, but the margin for error shrinks considerably when you hit your 40s and beyond. At these ages your body can no longer absorb the shock of a box of Krispy Kreme doughnuts or a pint of Ben & Jerry's without experiencing some damage.

I will later describe a dietary lifestyle that will help you not only shed unwanted pounds, but also calm inflammation, lower stress, give you more energy, help you sleep better, and smooth out the midlife hormonal roller coaster you're currently riding. The effort is worth it! When you know these secrets you can age beautifully and flow gracefully through your senior years.

How is Your Thyroid?

Many women develop hypothyroidism (an underactive thyroid) during or after pregnancy, or during perimenopause or menopause, due to hormonal changes. This problem can be confusing as symptoms of hypothyroidism and menopause often overlap with each other. Doctors who pass off these symptoms as a normal "change of life" will not correctly diagnose this disease. I'll lead you through the ins and outs of this very common disorder and what to do about it. If you know already that you have an underactive thyroid, I will guide you through the most common causes as outlined by Dr. Kharrazian in *Why Do I Still Have Thyroid Symptoms?*

Has Your Immunity Gone Haywire?

Functional medicine shines when it comes to identifying chronic "mystery" disorders that make standard health care doctors shrug their shoulders and write a script for Prozac. Being told that you have a "mystery" disorder is a huge clue that your doctor may not be up to date on the latest research, because researchers have uncovered many so-called health mysteries in the last decade. In fact, it's an exciting time in health care for practitioners lucky enough to study under professionals such as Datis Kharrazian, who takes the time to read all the latest studies, talk to researchers, distill the information into clinically valid applications, and teach practitioners like myself.

Functional medicine practitioners now know that nine times out of ten, "mystery" is code for "autoimmune." **When you have a condition that is persistent, seemingly irresolvable, and seems to flare up with no rhyme or reason, there's a strong possibility you have an autoimmune condition.** This means your immune system has gone haywire and is attacking and destroying the very thing it was designed to protect – your body. Some of the more commonly known autoimmune diseases are Type 1 diabetes, Hashimoto's disease, psoriasis, and multiple sclerosis. However, you can develop an autoimmune reaction to anything in your body – any tissue, enzyme, or hormone. Autoimmunity can be pretty complex at times, and pretty straightforward at others.

Some women know they have an autoimmune or inflammatory disorder because their doctor has made this diagnosis. Most commonly it is Hashimoto's disease. However, many more people suffer from an autoimmune reaction, which is different than a full-blown disease, and they don't know it. Instead, they suffer from mysterious symptoms, such as fatigue, and don't know why.

Medical doctors can't diagnose an autoimmune disease or code it for insurance until it has destroyed most of a particular tissue or gland. For instance, a person can suffer for years with symptoms similar to multiple sclerosis, Addison's disease, Type 1 diabetes, or other conditions before enough tissue has been damaged for a doctor to be able to diagnose it based on symptoms and testing. In the meantime you're hung out to dry or told you suffer from a psychological problem. This is also partly because traditional medicine can do very little to treat chronic autoimmune and inflammatory disorders, or reduce the associated symptoms of constant pain, fatigue, or other complaints. Fortunately, in functional medicine we can run lab tests that tell you if an autoimmune reaction is causing your symptoms, and also give you the dietary and nutritional tools to significantly improve how you feel and function.

Is Your Blood Sugar Out of Balance?

When you were a kid, did you ever set up a bunch of dominos in a long, curving line and then gently tip the first one over to watch in delight as all the dominoes behind it fell in a long cascade? When it comes to poor health, imbalanced blood sugar is often the first domino that pushes down all the other ones behind it. The other fallen dominoes are usually fatigue (due to insulin resistance), low cortisol levels, low progesterone, or a leaky gut. Together we'll explore the answer to the question, how did this happen to me? I'll show you the basics of blood sugar and what to do to stabilize it, regain your strength, and get back your mojo.

Are Your Adrenal Glands Fatigued?

Another major player in the puzzle of why you may be tired is your adrenal function. The adrenal glands, which sit atop the kidneys, secrete hormones to help keep the body balanced despite life's daily stressors. Unfortunately, daily stress can sometimes feel like an all-out assault these days. By the time many of us hit midlife, our adrenal glands have been overworked and are fried. This is what can make perimenopause and menopause traumatic for so many women.

As the ovaries wind down and produce less estrogen and progesterone, the adrenal glands produce these hormones instead to gently ease us into our golden years. But when the adrenal glands are in total burn out from years of abuse and overuse, producing reproductive hormones falls to the bottom of the to-do list, somewhere after "keep body alive, upright, and walking." As a result, hormone function goes into a tailspin. I'll show you how to determine the current functioning of your adrenal glands and what to do to improve it.

Do You Take Good Care of Your Brain?

People often ignore the importance of their brain health. It's imperative to learn how to properly feed and care for your brain, especially at a time of life when memory loss is a viable threat. Now is your time to shine in your career, start a new business, or step up your game in other important areas. Don't let an ignored or ailing brain stand in the way.

It's also important to know that estrogen profoundly affects how well your brain operates, so we'll discuss how to buffer the consequences of fluctuating or declining hormones. I'll teach you more about how nurturing your most precious organ profoundly improves your health and happiness. Many clients tell me that while they may look the same on the outside, in their mind they know they are "not thinking right." Where did I set the keys down? Where did I park the car? What's that person's name again? Then they start feeling like this confusion and fogginess must be something they're imagining or a normal aspect of aging.

We will be looking at the hormone-brain relationship, how oxygen, blood sugar levels, gluten sensitivity, and neurotransmitters affect intelligence, optimism, and confidence. There are science-based, proven answers to these nagging issues, solutions that will prevent and stop the progression of feeling as though you are losing your mind.

Do You Know How Your Evolving Environment Affects Your Health?

I will also explore the relatively new and very real effects of environmental toxins and electro smog –from cell phones, cell towers, Wi-Fi, and electrical appliances – on your health and hormonal balance. The seriousness of the impact of these devices on our health is similar to how germs were initially viewed. Many people didn't believe that germ theory was real because germs couldn't be easily seen. An increasing number of studies are exposing the threat to our health from many advances in modern technology; I'll share with you how to protect yourself and help buffer the damage from these unavoidable external influences.

How Functional Medicine Creates Lasting Change

One of the biggest differences between functional protocols and pharmaceutical-based medicine is that functional protocols don't apply a 'quick fix' through pills or surgery. Sure, sometimes a particular supplement ends up being the magic bullet, but those are the unusual cases. Usually healing involves making lifestyle changes through focused work and determination. Although it's not as easy as taking a pill, functional medicine offers much safer, more effective, long-term solutions.

After a period of adaptation to a new diet and protocol, the changes in your body feel really good, and you begin to naturally desire healthier foods and daily physical activity. An elegant system for healing is already built into the body and begging to shine. Feed your body the right foods; nudge it in the right direction with specific herbs and supplements, free it through physical activity, and it will leap into action for you.

I believe the human body is the physical embodiment of unconditional love. No matter how badly you have treated your body in the past, it serves endlessly because it loves you; it exists to carry you on your life journey and desires nothing more than to please you. However, being a biological organism, it has needs (similar to a faithful pet!) and requires proper care, feeding, attention, and love. I'll share with you the tools needed to nurture your body back to excellent health so it can continue its mission of serving you and giving physical form to your soul. Don't be a prisoner in your own body; let it express you fully and in all your greatness.

How Functional Medicine Lab Tests Are Different

In functional medicine we use quite a bit of lab testing. Saliva, blood, and stool testing are the "gold standards." This careful analysis of your body removes guesswork and 'shots in the dark,' and follow-up testing can confirm that changes to your diet or lifestyle are on the right track. Lab testing will shed considerable light on the causes of your symptoms and provide a starting point from which to recover your missing mojo. Armed with information about what's causing your symptoms, you then know which recommended science-based nutrition and lifestyle changes are the best choices to get you started on your healing journey.

"But I've already done lab tests out the wazoo!" you exclaim. In functional medicine we do labs differently. For one thing, we order more complete and thorough testing. When screening for a thyroid problem, for instance, most doctors in the regular medical model order just one or two blood markers or tests such as TSH (thyroid stimulating hormone). The reason for this is that it's less expensive to run just one or two markers instead of a complete thyroid panel that has 6 or 7 markers. Unfortunately, this really doesn't give you the "why" of what's causing the thyroid issue. Dr. Kharrazian identified 22 patterns of low thyroid function, and only one responds to thyroid medication. So, some people will be identified as having a low thyroid by just running the TSH marker. But if you're not one of them, you will continue to struggle with your health. You won't have all the pieces of the puzzle. In functional medicine we look at a half-dozen different markers, because we know multiple factors may contribute to hypothyroidism, which saps you of energy, joy, hair, and sex drive. (See appendix for information on the blood work protocols I use most often with my patients.)

In addition, most doctors flag only the results that are outside the more broadened "reference ranges" on your blood report when interpreting lab tests. These standard lab ranges are not useful for two reasons. One is that they only screen for pathological disease. For example, a wide lab reference range will declare that your blood sugar is normal until you develop diabetes, or that your thyroid level is normal until you have full-blown thyroid disease. So the gland or organ has to be in a critical state before it is considered an issue with these broadened reference ranges. Trouble could be brewing, but the particular test is not being flagged. You feel a false sense of security that all is well. This can leave you vulnerable to waiting for things to get better, or worse, believing that "maybe it is all in my head."

The second reason standard lab ranges have limited usefulness is because they are based on the results of all the people who visited that lab in the last year. This means the definition of healthy and unhealthy hinges on the people who had their blood drawn there, and presumably this was done because most of the people getting tested were not feeling well. This explains why your doctor runs labs and tells you the results are "normal" when you can barely get up to use the toilet, much less clean it. As our population gets sicker and sicker, then "ill" will become the new "normal!" But you are being told all is well because these expanded reference ranges are not flagging the problem. I look at both "schools of thought," which tells us a story of the true condition of your blood work.

With functional protocols, we have our own set of ranges based on comparing your blood levels to the levels in *healthy people.* **We use ranges that will identify a trend toward disease that can be caught and reversed before it's too late.** We also pay attention to what reference ranges would be "flagged" in the traditional medical model and compare them to the ranges we use all across the country in functional protocols, so that we stay up-to-date on trends in the traditional healthcare system. If you just look at the traditional reference ranges, you don't get a true picture of your health status. You might be told that your glucose is fine, when it is not. With the functional medicine ranges you can start making lifestyle changes to correct issues before they become pathological.

The Power of a Positive Outlook in Rebuilding Health

Although functional medicine has made significant inroads into the management of chronic health conditions, this doesn't mean functional medicine is omnipotent. There is still so much we don't know. One piece of the puzzle we know very little about is your attitude. There are subconscious forces at work we practitioners can't always get a handle on, ethereal emotional, psychological, and energetic forces that lie outside the nuts-and-bolts of physiology, which is the domain of functional medicine. It's not uncommon to see better outcomes in patients who have a positive outlook than in those who cling to an angry, defeatist, or negative attitude. We know that these forces can have a powerful positive impact on our health.

I know it is hard to stay positive when you feel like "road kill" all the time, but spending even a few minutes each day doing positive self-talk, positive visualization, or prayer and meditation has been proven to improve the ability to cope and to heal. I will return to this topic again later in the book.

The take away message is that if your labs are normal but you feel "at the end of your rope," questioning why you're still alive, then your health is most definitely not normal. You are not well. You were designed to be vibrant, curious, and engaged in life, to feel and express joy, and to exist in a state of positive well-being more days than not. Perimenopause and menopause are not the end of the road, or the beginning of a descent into poor health. With the right information and tools under your belt, this stage of life can be a glorious new beginning to your second act.

This is not a get-well-quick scheme. It is a revolutionary approach that takes dedication and persistence. For best results you have to want this; you have to want to feel better, to take back your health, and regain the mojo of your younger years. I can tell you that the results are more than worth the effort. It was worth it to me personally. I have been thrilled and astounded to watch the remarkable shifts in so many clients who wanted this, and I look forward to those shifts happening in your health and how you think about your health, as we work together on the steps in this book.

*Fasten your seat belts ThyroSisters;
we have embarked on an exciting journey together.
Some of the principles that I am about to share
with you are very different than what you are
used to hearing or doing, which may create a
paradigm shift in your thinking. That is what I hope
will happen as you read this book.*

CHAPTER 2
THE OVER-ZEALOUS PUZZLE PIECE: Is Your Immune System Attacking Itself?

If you struggle with mysterious and chronic symptoms, yet all your lab tests are normal, you may have an autoimmune reaction in which the body attacks its own cells, tissues, and organs. The hormonal fluctuations of pregnancy, perimenopause, and menopause can trigger autoimmunity. The confusing symptoms of an autoimmune response are not identifiable on standard lab testing, leaving you stranded in despair, because traditional medical treatments can't help you.

Autoimmunity is one of the most common health conditions today, dwarfing heart disease and cancer combined (American Autoimmune Related Diseases Association I., 2004-2014). So why does it get so little attention? Because short of prescribing steroids or surgically removing the affected organ or tissue, conventional medicine doesn't have tools to help and just throws up its hands. In fact, due to how prevalent autoimmunity is, if you have chronic, undiagnosed symptoms, the chances are good that you have an autoimmune condition and have not been properly diagnosed or told how to effectively manage your condition.

What is Autoimmunity?

Autoimmunity is when your immune system, which is designed to protect your body, goes haywire and begins attacking your body instead. Your immune cells mistakenly recognize different proteins—organs, body tissue, hormones, neurotransmitters, and enzymes—as harmful invaders and attack and destroy them. Once the immune system identifies a protein as an invader, it tags it with antibodies for permanent recognition, like stamping it with a barcode that can be scanned later for identification.

Examples of autoimmune disorders include Hashimoto's disease (attack on the thyroid gland), multiple sclerosis (loss of nerve function), Type I diabetes (attack on cells in the pancreas), alopecia (hair loss), vitiligo (patches of skin that lose color), and pernicious anemia (B12 anemia).

Autoimmunity is considered a permanent condition. However, if you're willing to step out of the mainstream medical paradigm, the good news is that functional medicine offers many effective ways for taming autoimmune attacks, and even forcing them into remission.

You Could Have Autoimmunity and Not Know it

The biggest problem with autoimmunity is when someone appears to have an autoimmune reaction but imaging scans come back showing no abnormalities, lab tests are normal, or the symptoms are not advanced enough for medical diagnosis. A very important aspect of autoimmunity that Dr. Kharrazian describes in his book, *Why Isn't My Brain Working?* is that you can have an autoimmune reaction without having an autoimmune disease. Symptoms can actually be quite severe and the condition fairly advanced, but it is not technically a disease until the particular marker for that autoimmune is formally diagnosed on a blood panel. If your doctor doesn't check for autoimmune markers, you will never be diagnosed.

The sad news is that a person can suffer from autoimmune reactions for years, decades, or even a lifetime with no diagnosis, no medical explanation, and no help. Many people, especially those with Hashimoto's hypothyroidism, are dismissed, ignored, and even

belittled by doctors for complaining about symptoı
have no explanation. Or they are inappropriately pı   H
antidepressants to treat these mysterious, worsenin;

Luckily, today we have advanced testing th;
whether you suffer from autoimmunity. **Cyrex Lat**
immunity laboratory specializing in immunology and
autoimmunity, effectively screens for the 24 most common forms
of autoimmune reactions with just one test. The results may not
only explain your mystery symptoms, but also alert you to
autoimmune reactions you were not even aware of. For example, you
may be experiencing autoimmune attacks against brain or nerve
tissue that could predispose you to multiple sclerosis or other
medical conditions years down the road. Or you may have
autoimmunity affecting joint tissue that could debilitate you later in
life, even though you currently experience little to no pain. By
learning whether you have an autoimmune reaction early with the
right testing, you can use functional medicine principles to treat your
symptoms and prevent the onset of a full-blown disease later in life.

Restoring Immune System Balance

If you discover that you have an autoimmune disease, such as
Hashimoto's, it is important to understand how your immune system
now perceives itself. For example, let's say that your immune system
is a huge Boston Red Sox fan, which means that it hates the New
York Yankees with a vengeance! Yankee fans tend to wear navy
blue ball caps, so your immune system decides to attack anyone
wearing a navy blue baseball cap. Then here comes your thyroid,
minding its own business, proudly wearing a navy blue San Diego
Padres cap. Your immune system can't tell the difference between
the Yankees hat and the Padres hat. All it sees is a navy blue cap,
which means ATTACK!

When someone has Hashimoto's disease, their immune
system often attacks the thyroid, which results in lower functioning,
less thyroid hormone, and all the lousy symptoms that make you feel
like you're falling apart.

When you have Hashimoto's, you don't just have a "thyroid"
problem, you have an "autoimmune" problem. This is an important
distinction, because the thyroid hormones that doctors commonly
prescribe to hypothyroid patients do nothing to manage the

.imoto's. All they do is mask the symptoms (and leave out an .portant piece of the puzzle) by providing your body with synthetic thyroid. If you have a leak in your gas tank, adding more gas will help your car keep running, but it won't fix the leak!

To find the source of your thyroid problem, we often have to look deeper. Dr. Datis Kharrazian introduced the concept of TH1 and TH2, two kinds of immune "T-helper" cells. These immune cells should balance each other, sort of like a teeter-totter with kids of equal weight on either side. TH1 is the part of your immune system that reacts immediately to an invader, such as a virus or a splinter. In the case of a splinter, it creates swelling, redness, and pus. TH2 is the part that tags the invader with antibodies so it knows to destroy and remove the invader in the future. An example is developing antibodies to a virus through exposure, either from a vaccine or a virus such as chicken pox.

If your immune system is out of balance because of stress— physical, chemical, or emotional—either TH1 or TH2 will become dominant, predisposing you to autoimmunity. Or to say it another way, if one child on the teeter-totter grows bigger, the smaller child is stranded at the top and can't do its job in your body. There are specific blood tests that determine if one or the other of these immune cell types is dominant. This information is useful, because by stimulating the weaker cells we can help restore balance to the immune system, and calm or halt autoimmune attacks. We can also do a "TH1/TH2 challenge," using herbs or supplements to stimulate either TH1 or TH2, and monitor how you respond.

Support TH3 for Better Immune Balance

Regardless of whether you are TH1 or TH2 dominant, you want to support another immune player called TH3. The job of TH3 is to call off an immune reaction so neither TH1 nor TH2 gets out of control, much like a mom refereeing a squabble: "OK, both you kids are in time out." Fortunately, supporting TH3 isn't difficult.

Compounds that support TH3 and help dampen inflammation include vitamin D, Omega-3, and glutathione (an essential antioxidant). Oral glutathione doesn't work because the stomach acid eats it up, but certain nutritional compounds, such as N-acetyl L-cysteine, can raise your glutathione levels

Chronic inflammation of the blood vessels plays a major role in the initiation and progression of degenerative diseases such as cardiovascular disease, atherosclerosis, and autoimmune. I like to run multiple biomarkers for heart muscle (NT-proBNP and cTnl), along with inflammatory biomarkers (IL-6,IL-17A, TNF-a,Lp-PLA2, and hs-CRP). These markers are known to become elevated in patients with various stages of degenerative diseases (www.ThyroSisters.com provides information on how you can be tested for these cutting-edge biomarkers.)

It is so important to test and not guess about your inflammation status. The Omega-3 Index is the result of Dr. William Harri's 30-year research on fatty acids and cardiovascular disease. It provides a measure of omega-fatty acids, EPA+DHA, in red blood cells, which also relates to risk for heart disease. You can find more information about this test at www.ThyroSisters.com

Dampen TH17 to Tame Autoimmunity

While TH3 helps put the brakes on TH dominance, TH17 does the opposite: *it fuels an autoimmune attack.* TH17 is bad news since it leads to tissue damage. The original function of TH17 cells is to protect the body against bacteria and fungi, and to help recruit, activate, and help migration of neutrophils. Neutrophils are the most common type of white blood cell, and are the first immune cells to arrive at a site of infection. A lack of TH 17 cells leaves you susceptible to opportunistic infections. But like good girls gone wild, TH17 causes inflammation in an autoimmune disease such as Hashimoto's, which in turn causes tissue damage. (L, 2007)

The most effective way to dampen TH17 is to take therapeutic doses of curcumin and resveratrol. You may be familiar with curcumin as a culinary spice; it is responsible for the yellow color of Indian curry and American mustard. It is delicious and will spice up your foods while spicing up your health. Curcumin is found in Turmeric, which is derived from the rhizomes (underground stems) of the plant Curcuma longa, a member of the ginger family. Curcumin has powerful antioxidant and anti-inflammatory properties, and is the most active part of turmeric. I use an emulsified liquid curcumin that delivers a whopping 420 mg per teaspoon, sometimes three times a day depending on the application. It also contains black pepper extract to enhance absorption. This is very important because without the black pepper extract, or piperine, there is very little absorption. Be patient my sweet friends, lab studies show that it takes about eight weeks to notice the full effects of decreased inflammation, especially micro-inflammation in the GI tract associated with inflammatory bowel disease.

I also recommend taking an emulsified liquid resveratrol, together with the turmeric formula. Resveratrol is found naturally in the skin of grapes and acts as an antioxidant and anti-inflammatory. Red wine contains resveratrol, but it would take a boatload of red wine to derive the benefits of resveratrol, so it's better to take it in capsule form (life doesn't seem fair sometimes, does it?) Resveratrol has been found to lower blood sugar and LDL, the bad cholesterol. One teaspoon delivers 250 mg. Although curcumin and resveratrol are highly effective when taken alone, studies show they work even better when taken together (Sharma S, 2007).

Glutathione Can Help

One of your biggest allies in the battle against autoimmune attacks is glutathione, the body's master antioxidant. **Glutathione is the body's most important antioxidant because it is made within the cell.** It is the biggest "muscle-man" on the beach. Other better known, but not as strong, muscle men antioxidants are vitamins C and E. These powerhouse antioxidant players are important because they neutralize free radicals, but glutathione wins the muscle man contest for strength, endurance and detoxification. Your body produces glutathione all the time. But stress, pollution, poor eating habits, and trauma deplete your supply of this molecule, making Mr. Atlas look like a poisoned puppy.

Glutathione has three simple proteins: cysteine, glycine, and glutamine. It contains a sulfur group, which is critical for immune function, controlling inflammation, preventing disease, and aging well. Examples of glutathione or sulfur rich foods are garlic, onions, broccoli, kale, cabbage, walnuts, and lamb. They are all high in N-acetyl cysteine, alpha lipoic acid, vitamin B6 and B12, and selenium, which are important for the production and recycling of glutathione. Glutathione helps shield the body not only from autoimmune attacks, but also from environmental toxins. Glutathione is critical to cell survival and DNA repair, plays a role in eliminating heavy metals, and, most importantly, helps regulate the immune system. Many cells in the body produce glutathione, but most of it is produced in the liver. When the body is deficient in glutathione, many health disorders can result, including autoimmunity. So we want this muscle man flexing on the beach of our lives forever. No weaklings in our Mojo tribe!

Taking a glutathione supplement (unless it's S-acetyl glutathione) isn't effective because the stomach breaks the chemical down, limiting its absorption. Instead, it works best to take compounds that boost glutathione; the most effective are N-acetyl L-cysteine, alpha lipoic acid, cordyceps, gotu kola, selenium, milk thistle, glutamic acid, and glycine. I also use an oral liquid – liposomal glutathione – that is absorbed through the stomach lining before being subjected to digestion.

Gluten: The Autoimmune Connection

Now, through this process I want you to be very kind to yourself. You are entering a new season of your life; you are making great strides. One of these strides is recognizing that you are worthy and valuable. Spark a reconnection with yourself. No more self-hatred, or "should have," "could have," "would have" thinking. It's in the past. It's not important how many times you failed, but how many times you got back up again. I would like you to approach this next subject with abundance, not deprivation. You haven't done anything wrong by not sticking to a strict diet your whole life. In fact, I feel that perpetual dieting creates self-loathing, but I will talk more about that later.

If you have an autoimmune reaction, you need to give up gluten for good. I don't mean to sound harsh, but it's that simple, and that effective. Gluten (a protein found in many grains) is the most common trigger for autoimmunity. **Research has linked gluten with 55 different diseases, and the majority are autoimmune conditions.**

What the heck is this gluten thing anyway, and why has it become public enemy number one? (I know I am going to go into the Post Office one day and see a poster hanging on the wall titled MOST WANTED, with a picture of a grain of wheat!) Remember when you were a kid and you could smell biscuits or waffles cooking? Or look forward to eating delicious pasta at your favorite

Italian restaurant? You might have driven past fields of amber waves of grain blowing in the breeze.

Well it looks, tastes, and smells the same, but now the seed that goes into the ground is made from a CHEMICAL, not a real seed that God made. White flour, oats, barley, wheat, and rye are made from these seeds. Most of the above mentioned grains in the US are from genetically modified seeds from Monsanto and your body does not recognize them as real food! In an effort to serve you, your body starts to inflame against what is perceived as a toxin, in order to get rid of it. You might feel cranky, brain fog, or bloated. You may have digestive issues or can't lose weight. Your symptoms come and go and you chalk it up to age or menopause. You don't really put together that gluten and your symptom are related. The months and years go on. You have been eating gluten all this time, and some straw breaks the camel's back. The digestion/elimination gets worse; you don't want to go out in public due to extreme flatulence (cutting the cheese, as my sisters would say). You have three different sizes of clothes in the closet, partly due to your gut being so inflamed and leaking toxins. You can't lose weight, even living on whole grain dry toast and organic raw milk, and walking every day.

Oh and by the way, our digestive tract has its own nervous system called the enteric system, and it's not connected to the rest of the nervous system. You are not aware that you are inflamed, you have no fever, no swelling, no real objective findings to associate gluten with your fatigue, weight gain, insomnia, constipation or diarrhea, or why you can't remember where you parked the car after being in the store for 5 minutes.

The brain and the nervous system are most commonly affected by intolerance to gluten. Because the brain is so adept at compensating for problems, you can go years, or decades, not knowing that autoimmunity is present in your body, or brushing off symptoms of brain fog, memory loss, or poor balance, while your risk of developing dementia, Alzheimer's disease, Parkinson's disease, multiple sclerosis, or other neurological disorders significantly increases. (Benkler M, 2009), (Levin M, 2002), (Perlmutter, 2013). This is partly due to inflammation of the microglia cells of the brain. Dr. Kharrizan has a saying: "leaky gut, leaky brain." The connection between gluten intolerance and celiac disease (an autoimmune disease triggered by gluten) and the hypothyroidism that is the result of Hashimoto's disease, is well established (Barton SH, 2008). **I recommend a gluten-free diet for all my patients with Hashimoto's; many experience dramatic improvement simply by taking this step.**

Eliminating gluten in the diet stops the progression of the disease, and then through science-based nutrition we can balance and repair the damage that has already been done. (If the idea of giving up all of your gluten-infused foods has you clutching your cookies and pasta for dear life, it really isn't as hard or painful as you imagine. I will guide you to a better, gluten-free diet in Chapter Ten.)

Standard tests for gluten sensitivity fail to successfully diagnose many people. This is because the tests only assess one gluten protein called "alpha gliadin." Researchers at Cyrex Labs have identified 12 different gluten proteins, and they test for sensitivity to all of them. Also, standard celiac tests only detect an autoimmune reaction in the gut by checking for antibodies to intestinal transglutaminase (an enzyme used as a celiac marker), but Cyrex Labs can identify transglutaminase antibodies to the skin, and neurological tissue triggered by gluten, since you can have celiac disease that affects your skin or your brain, rather than your gut.

What's the simple way to know if gluten is friend or foe? Stop eating it for 6 weeks, and see how you feel. Then slowly introduce wheat, or wheat germ, faro, semolina, spelt, kamut, rye, barley or triticale back into your diet. I want you to live big and abundantly! I am not suggesting going without your favorite pasta dish or cereal, just use gluten-free brands made from non-GMO corn, brown rice, or potatoes. Supermarkets have gluten-free flours to bake with, also pasta, salad dressings, and condiments.

Going Beyond Gluten

Sometimes, banishing gluten from your diet will dramatically reduce or eliminate your autoimmune symptoms, but you may also need to eliminate other foods. In my experience the more severe the autoimmune reaction, the more foods the person may need to eliminate. Now, having said that, please know that you are going to have plenty to eat, and not go hungry. You're not going to be one of those health nuts that can't eat anything, living on wheat grass shots.

But the next most common food people often need to stop consuming is dairy, which includes butter, cheese, yogurt, and other milk products. Eggs are inflammatory to some people. Some other problematic foods you may want to temporarily remove from your diet are soy, lectins (which are in grains and beans), nightshades (potatoes, tomatoes, eggplants, and peppers), and polysaccharides (long-chain sugars in grains, legumes, and all sweeteners except honey). Some people react to foods that seem unlikely, such as bananas. Experiment with your diet (or get tested for possible sensitivities to these foods) and find out exactly what your body loves and what you can eliminate to rebuild that much-needed mojo!

At this point you may be thinking, "This sounds very boring, and limited. This isn't how I want to live my life!" Keep in mind that the point is not to deprive you, but to greatly enhance your life, your health and how you feel. Now I will introduce you to colorful, beautiful, gracious ways to eat and age with vitality. Embrace the ideas in these books and add your own.

Kris Carr's *Crazy Sexy Diet* overflows with delicious whole-food recipes. Read and be inspired by her courageous and inspiring story of living for over 10 years with cancer in remission. Another wonderful resource is *Break the Sugar Habit in 21 Days* by Lee Milteer. Bless your food for sustaining you; thank your body for serving you all these years. Even if you are fighting a health challenge or have a few extra love handles to lose, love and be grateful for your body. We are looking for progress not perfection. This is a marathon not a sprint. Be patient and pay attention to how you feel when you eat specific foods. Keeping a journal or food diary helps.

Although we have many tools in our autoimmune management toolkit, your diet will be one of the most important and powerful. As I will discuss later, an elimination/provocation diet, or testing for food sensitivities using the Cyrex Labs food sensitivity panel will help identify which foods provoke your immune system. Look at this as going on an adventure. Look at your hormone or thyroid auto immune challenge as a gift. Know that you are gaining in knowledge and wisdom, and be proud of yourself for taking control of your body and health.

This is a fresh, clean, and empowering way to eat and to live. It will take a little time to adjust to new ways of eating and thinking, but be kind to yourself as you do so. You are not alone, always remember that, okay? You have tackled obstacles before, and by the grace of God, you have come a long way. Your suffering will lessen, you will shine again soon. You are learning to eat clean, to keep your temple body moving. Pray, laugh, lose the stinkin' thinkin' and ignite that former spark of your beautiful life.

Living with Hashimoto's Disease

If you're a woman with autoimmunity, there's a good chance that you have the autoimmune thyroid condition known as Hashimoto's disease, which causes low thyroid function, also called hypothyroidism. **Hashimoto's is the most common cause of hypothyroidism in the United States and affects up to 10 percent of the population** (Hollowell JG, 2002). Graves' disease, an autoimmune disorder that causes hyperthyroidism, is less common.

It's also common for women with Hashimoto's to develop additional autoimmune reactions to other tissues in the body, and to then develop conditions such as pernicious anemia, Type 1 diabetes, or vitiligo (a skin pigment condition). Also, Hashimoto's has associated symptoms that often overlap with menopausal symptoms, such as depression, fatigue, weight gain, or insomnia. This is why I order the appropriate lab tests that will pinpoint the primary culprit. When a woman has thyroid-related or menopausal symptoms, treating a menopausal condition with thyroid medications, or a thyroid condition with hormone therapy, can be ineffective or even worsen symptoms. For example, giving a women thyroid medication when she may have Hashimoto's can create inflammation which reflects as weight gain (Cooper, 2012).

How Does Autoimmunity Affect Hormones?

Most often autoimmunity affects perimenopause and menopause symptoms indirectly. **Autoimmune reactions are severe stressors for the body and will throw your adrenal function out of balance.** The stress will also promote leaky gut and general inflammation in the body. You may have heard the term "leaky gut" before. This is when the tight junctions of your intestinal tract break open and toxins such as parasites, viruses, and bacteria leak out into your bloodstream (I know, yuck).

These invaders start circulating through your bloodstream instead of staying in the intestines and being excreted through fecal matter, urine, or sweat. This causes our old enemy, inflammation (more about how you can counteract and prevent this later). These factors will, in turn, zap hormone balance and set you up for the severe symptoms sometimes associated with menopause.

However, there are times when autoimmunity directly affects the reproductive system. An autoimmune reaction against the adrenal glands, which is more common than we initially thought (National Endocrine and Metabolic Diseases Information Service, 2009), can leave the adrenal glands too impaired to take over hormone production as the ovaries wind down during menopause. Serious adrenal autoimmunity is called Addison's disease; many people have adrenal autoimmunity without it escalating to the point of becoming a disease. Women can also have autoimmune reactions against their ovaries, or against estrogen or progesterone. This response not only leads to infertility but also causes menopausal symptoms.

As you can see, there is far more to menopausal symptoms than just progesterone, estrogen, and testosterone. While these sex hormones are important, in this chapter you have learned how an undiagnosed autoimmune disorder could be wreaking havoc on your health and "mimicking" the traditional symptoms that often lead to the recommendation for hormone replacement.

Secrets Whispered to a ThyroSister

Clients often ask how they developed their autoimmune condition. The research suggests a genetic predisposition triggered by environmental factors (American Autoimmune Related Diseases Association I., 2004-2014). Just because you have the genes for a disease doesn't mean you will get it. But a lifetime of poor diet, too much stress, imbalanced blood sugar, chronic inflammation, and environmental toxins can trigger autoimmunity.

* Curcumin is a spice that is the active component of turmeric. Add a tablespoon of olive oil to 500-1,000mg of curcumin for better absorption. Curcumin protects the liver, stimulates the gallbladder, and is a powerful antioxidant. Curcumin also enhances the effectiveness of other important supplements such as resveratrol and quercetin.

* Visit our website (www.ThyroSisters.com) for a *symptom survey* to help you determine what your symptoms might mean, particularly in relation to a possible autoimmune reaction.

* Test, don't guess. A multiple tissue antibody panel can reveal whether autoimmune reactions are causing your symptoms. Go to www.ThyroSisters.com to find out more about this and other available tests.

* Test for which foods cross-react with gluten or cause sensitivity with the Gluten-Associated Cross-Reactive Foods and Foods Sensitivity panel (you can find these at www.ThyroSisters.com). Once you understand which foods your body can't tolerate, take them out of your diet. Foods that trigger your immune system, such as gluten, constantly cause autoimmunity to flare. You also need to remove other "trigger foods" from your diet, which may include dairy, eggs, soy, nuts, or other grains. Cross reactive Foods and Foods Sensitivity panel (www.cyrex.labs.com).

CHAPTER 3
THE OVERWORKED PUZZLE PIECE:
Is Your Thyroid Out of Gas?

> **"** I was too old for a paper route, too young for social security and too tired for an affair. **"**
>
> *Erma Bombeck*

Fear gripped her voice, as her hands trembled.

"I am too tired to even go out to dinner, let alone cook it!" cried Katie, an attractive 48 year-old mother of two high school girls. "By 7:00 PM I feel exhausted, short tempered and cranky. I have been trying to take off 10 pounds forever with no luck. I get up in the middle of the night once or twice, and then my mind goes on over-drive over nothing. I have a low libido, I feel stressed over little things." Like many of my patients, doctors had told Katie there was nothing wrong with her, but she knew something was wrong. "I don't think it is my thyroid, I had it checked. It's normal. I just don't 'feel like myself.'" Unfortunately, it's a story I've heard far too often. "I feel foggy and anxious. I over-think the most mundane decisions. And I fear everything: fear of financial failure, fear the kids won't get into the right schools, fear of what people think of me, fear my health is going to be like this forever, fear of loneliness, fear of fear." Katie put her head in her hands. "I used to be confident, decisive, and full of vitality for my husband and my life."

These fast-paced times leave us ladies tired—tired from long days at work and coming home to care for kids, cook dinner, and do the housework. Tired from diets that harm our bodies, lack of sleep, too little play, and environmental toxins. After a while, all these factors take their toll on our bodies, and rare is the woman who escapes unscathed. For women like Katie, a hard-hit gland is the thyroid, and many women develop hypothyroidism, an underactive thyroid gland.

As if life wasn't tiring enough under normal circumstances, when your thyroid falters you become even more tired, in addition to feeling depressed, cold, lethargic, and foggy-brained. Getting through daily life with symptoms of low thyroid activity requires mountains of pure will and stamina. Life should not be this hard, and it doesn't have to be.

Many women find that their perimenopause and menopausal symptoms, weight gain, and depression have more to do with their thyroid faltering than with decreasing hormones. Symptoms can overlap, so if you feel lousy, low thyroid function, whether due to autoimmune thyroid disease (called Hashimoto's after Dr. Hashimoto who first discovered this disease in the mid- forties) or another cause, needs to be ruled out.

Hashimoto's attacks the adrenals, digestive tract, blood sugar levels and the thyroid. Whether you have it can be determined by two blood variables called TPO and TGB (more about this later). Dr. Kharrizan, in his brilliance, discovered 22 patterns for low thyroid. To get to the root cause of your thyroid issues, and in turn ditch that fatigue, you need to know which pattern relates to your blood work. Do you have autoimmune Hashimoto's that is lowering your thyroid and wreaking havoc in the rest of your system? Or do you have primary low thyroid, not associated with Hashimoto's? Could it be that the pituitary gland is not working correctly? Or is the T4 hormone being released from the thyroid not converting to T3, which helps you think, metabolize, and sleep well? Is the gut not making enough neurotransmitters to trigger the hypothalamus, which triggers the pituitary to make TSH? Maybe the adrenals are not putting out enough cortisol to signal the hypothalamus/pituitary? There are 18 additional pathways that influence why you might have low thyroid. For a more in-depth discussion on this, pick up Dr. Kharrazian's book *Why Do I Still Have Thyroid Symptoms When My Labs Are Normal?*

Wheeeew! Are you getting tired just thinking about it? Well, don't fret, this is part of solving the puzzle, and perhaps why you have not found helpful answers in the past. There is more to getting to the root cause of your low thyroid than just checking TSH or taking your temperature in the morning.

If you are experiencing several of the following symptoms, I recommend getting a complete thyroid panel of blood tests to determine whether you suffer from an underactive thyroid disorder:

- **Fatigue**
- **Depression**
- **Constipation**
- **Cold hands and feet; very sensitive to cold weather**
- **Weight gain despite eating well and exercising**
- **Muscle cramps**
- **Frequently sick and recover slowly**
- **Wounds heal slowly**
- **Require excessive sleep to function**
- **Chronic digestive problems**
- **Dry skin and dry, brittle hair**
- **Cracked heels**
- **Hair loss**
- **Facial swelling**
- **Loss of outer eyebrows**
- **Low libido**

Paradoxically, some women with low thyroid function occasionally suffer from the symptoms of having too much thyroid hormone. This is because they have an autoimmune reaction against the thyroid gland. **Hashimoto's disease accounts for 90 percent of hypothyroid cases in the United States.** (Kharrazian D., 2010) This is a situation in which the immune system attacks the thyroid gland and destroys it, spilling excess thyroid hormone into the bloodstream and revving up the metabolism, making it look as though you have hyper or high thyroid.

ADDITIONAL SYMPTOMS OF A THYROID CONDITION:

Heart palpitations   **Increased pulse**

Trembling   **Insomnia**

Nervousness   **Night sweats**

Anxiety

When the body uses all of its energy just to cope with everyday life because thyroid function is low, other health problems may occur. For instance, I have seen many tired clients with fibromyalgia, and found that thyroid malfunction usually is involved at some level. **Since the thyroid gland controls metabolism, it is frequently involved when you feel tired all the time.**

But My Tests Are All Normal!

If you have already been to your doctor about thyroid concerns, he or she probably ordered only one thyroid blood test, the TSH (thyroid-stimulating hormone) test. What you may not know is that even though your doctor said your results were normal and pronounced you "fine," you may still have an underactive thyroid.

How can this be? Many conventional physicians still use the Thyroid Stimulating Hormone (TSH) EXPANDED range, of "normal" of 0.5 to 5.0, on the blood report. This causes you to think that you are within the normal guidelines and why you are being told everything is fine, that you are "normal" when you would be showing "abnormal" if the health care provider was using the range that was used for years in this country, which is 1.8 to 3.0.

So you can still be seen as "normal" in your doctor's eyes, but abnormal in terms of actual thyroid function. This explains why many women struggle with symptoms of low thyroid function (including extreme fatigue, weight gain, and hair loss), but are sent home from the doctor's office with no helpful information, and sometimes a prescription for Prozac.

44

If your doctor is testing you for hypothyroidism, ask to be tested for Hashimoto's disease too. Most conventional doctors don't test for it because they don't treat it any differently than hypothyroidism. However, functional medicine shines when it comes to managing autoimmune diseases, and we have many tools to help you manage your symptoms, even if you need thyroid hormones.

In addition to testing your TSH level, ask your doctor about a measure of two antibodies: thyroid peroxidase (TPO) and thyroglobulin (TGB) antibodies. If these tests come back positive, it means your immune system is attacking your thyroid, which is Hashimoto's disease. These tests usually cost less than $100, and the results are important for an accurate diagnosis. Proper treatment can radically improve your energy levels physically, mentally, emotionally, spiritually, and sexually.

If you do have an autoimmune condition you need to find out what is provoking the autoimmunity. A number of studies show a link between celiac disease or gluten intolerance, and Hashimoto's disease (Duntas, 2009). If you test positive for Hashimoto's disease, following a gluten-free diet is vital to help tame the autoimmune attacks and stop the progression. (We'll discuss eating for health in Part Two.)

Other triggers for autoimmunity include viral infection, bacteria (usually in the gut) parasites, mold, or fungus. Yikes, right? Hormone imbalances, blood sugar dysregulation, high cortisol, and chronic inflammation are other common conditions that can lead to an autoimmune disease. Periods of extreme stress, sleep deprivation, consuming excessive sugar or alcohol, an angry fight, and other stressors can trigger flare-ups of autoimmune disease as well. The good news is that there are solutions that will greatly improve how you feel. **Having an autoimmune disease really forces you to live a more balanced life and take careful care of your body.**

Clues Related to Thyroid Autoimmune Disease

Although lab testing is the only way to confirm an autoimmune disease, there are certain clues that help reveal whether you suffer from an autoimmune disease. One clue is that having one autoimmune disease (to include psoriasis, rheumatoid arthritis, ulcerative colitis, Sjögren's syndrome, scleroderma or lupus, or Type

1 diabetes) increases your risk of developing other autoimmune diseases. The combination of having an autoimmune condition and experiencing symptoms of hypothyroidism is a red flag to test for Hashimoto's disease. Also, failing to manage your autoimmune thyroid condition could set you up to develop additional autoimmune disorders.

In Katie's case, we ran a complete metabolic panel, a complete thyroid panel including antibodies, and a saliva cortisol test. The tests revealed that she had a low T3, high T4, and that her insulin was low before and after she ate. She was also anemic, had leaky gut, and had been combating a low grade chronic viral infection. She did not have Hashimoto's. Katie went on a special liquid glutathione, emulsified vitamin D, anti-inflammatory protein shakes, and a gluten free, organic diet. After 3 months she reported that her husband said she looked younger! She had lost 7 lbs, (she was still 10 lbs. over her goal weight), the sense of fear, anxiety, inner trembling, and stress had diminished. She was sleeping and had a renewed sense of "caring about the little things in life" to boot.

Before, Katie's symptoms had seemed insidious, always coming and going. She had started thinking things like, "Am I just imagining things? Am I just getting old?" **One of the ways you may recognize an autoimmune thyroid condition is if symptoms wax and wane.** This is because the immune system has periods of flare-up and remission. This explains why a woman with Hashimoto's disease can have symptoms of low thyroid function for a period of time, and then shift to symptoms of overly high thyroid function. She may need 12 hours of sleep one week and then can't get more than 3 hours of sleep the next. Or one week she feels depressed and lethargic, and the next she is a bundle of nerves and ready to jump out of her skin.

A third clue that an autoimmune condition may be lurking is when a patient has worked with many different practitioners and now takes an excessive number of different supplements. Although I work with supplements in my practice, I believe there is a limit. Your body on supplements is like an airplane gaining altitude: at first the plane needs a lot of fuel, but once it reaches cruising altitude less fuel is needed. At first there may be a little bit more "fuel," or supplements, needed but once you are on cruise control, you should not be taking a kitchen counter full of supplements.

In many cases the supplements a woman takes may be making her symptoms worse! For instance, immune stimulants such as echinacea or astragalus can make some people with autoimmunity problems significantly worse. Why? Because they fire up the dominant side of the immune system, causing even more inflammation. As in the previous teeter tooter example, these healthy substances make some people with autoimmune disease feel better and some worse, depending on if you are TH1 dominant or TH2 dominant (this can be determined by a blood test or elimination/provocation diet).

On the other hand you may feel better if the herb or supplement dampened down the overactive side of the immune system. This explains why your sister with an autoimmune disease can drink green tea and feels great, while you (who has an autoimmune), feels lousy no matter how many glasses you drink. Her immune system needs the green tea, while yours doesn't. This is just one example of why you need to test, and not guess. This is your precious life, so let's not take any chances about how you can get it back.

Another clue is noticing that your life and health seemed to fall apart after an illness, pregnancy, accident, divorce, death of a loved one, or some other major stressful event. Women who say they were never the same after having a baby or getting divorced sometimes have been to 12, 15, 20, or even 30 doctors and have a foot-tall stack of lab tests, because no one diagnosed their autoimmune condition, or was able to manage it effectively.

MAJOR THYROID AUTOIMMUNE TRIGGERS

- **Taking supplements containing iodine**
- **Undiagnosed anemia**
- **Unbalanced blood sugar**
- **High levels of prolactin**
- **Gluten sensitivity**
- **Vitamin D deficiency**
- **Impaired adrenal glands**
- **Leaky gut**

Thyroid Autoimmune Triggers

The following issues are the 'biggies' that can trigger or worsen thyroid autoimmune disorders. Review this list to search for additional clues to help you better understand what may be causing or contributing to your symptoms, how to evaluate for this condition, and what tools will help.

Be Wary of Iodine

I know there are several competing schools of thought on the following concept, and I now want to offer my thoughts and observations. The question is: can you correct thyroid problems with iodine? I especially have an appreciation for Dr. Brownstein's brilliant work on iodine and how important it is to everything from treating ADHD to improving the immune system. An iodine deficiency can cause hypothyroidism and goiter (enlarged thyroid). These conditions were common in the United States before the 1920s, which is why regular table salt is still commonly iodized, to combat these conditions (American Thryroid Association, 2014). But Iodine is not a cure-all for all thyroid conditions; it will solve thyroid problems that are caused by iodine deficiency. If that's not what's causing your thyroid to go haywire, you can actually worsen the problem by increasing iodine in your diet.

One of the biggest triggers for an autoimmune thyroid flare up is iodine. Dr. Kharrazian presents compelling research in his book, *Why Do I Still Have Thyroid Symptoms?* which shows how iodine promotes thyroid autoimmunity, and I have seen this connection in my clients and myself. If you have hypothyroid, without an autoimmune problem, then iodine supplementation may be just the answer. What is brought out in Dr. Kharrazian's work is that if you have Hashimoto's, it might be advantageous to supplement with 200 micrograms of selenium before introducing iodine. Selenium is a mineral found in the soil in most parts of the world. The best way to ingest selenium is through organic produce, and Brazil nuts. Only 3-4 Brazil nuts a day will give you a healthy thyroid hormone conversion.

Studies have shown that adequate selenium nutrition supports thyroid hormone synthesis and protects the thyroid gland from damage from excessive iodine exposure (Zimmermann MB, 2002). Another study found that selenium had an impact on inflammatory activity in thyroid-specific autoimmune disease; in reducing inflammation, selenium may reduce damage to thyroid tissue (Gartner R, 2002).

Selenium is also important in the conversion of T4 to T3, as the enzyme that removes iodine atoms from T4 during conversion is selenium dependent. T3 is the active form of thyroid hormone, and low T3 can cause hypothyroid symptoms. In cases of selenium deficiency, conversion of T4 to T3 is impaired, leading to hypothyroid symptoms (Miller JC1, 2012).

So the question remains, should you go off iodine, or should you go on selenium? The answer is, it depends! Connect with a functional health practitioner and test, don't guess. The best way to determine iodine status is through a diagnostic 24-hour urine loading test. This involves taking a large dose of iodine, and collecting urine for 24 hours afterwards. If you're iodine deficient, you'll retain more of the ingested iodine, and the level of iodine excreted will be lower.

Many supplements that claim to benefit the thyroid actually contain iodine. If you have Hashimoto's disease, you must avoid these. I realize iodine is very popular today and it can certainly have benefits, but for the person with Hashimoto's or even a family history of Hashimoto's, supplementing with iodine is not worth the risk.

Is Anemia Affecting Your Energy?

As a functional practitioner, I sometimes feel like a detective solving a mystery. Your symptoms and test results are clues, but as with all great mystery novels, there are unexpected twists and turns that thicken the plot or, as with your health, make finding the culprit difficult. A common plot twist in thyroid health is anemia. It's a little known, but quite common, issue that makes it difficult to tame an autoimmune condition.

Anemia is a medical condition in which the red blood cell count or hemoglobin is less than normal. In women, low hemoglobin means less than 12.0 gram/100ml. Iron is needed to make hemoglobin, a part of the red blood cells that acts like a taxicab for oxygen and carbon dioxide. It picks up oxygen in the lungs, drives it through the blood stream and drops it off in tissues like skin and muscles. Then, it picks up carbon dioxide and drives it back to the lungs where it is exhaled. Some women with anemia have no symptoms. Others may appear pale and feel weak or dizzy. Their hearts might race and they may get headaches. There are three main causes of anemia: blood loss, a low number of red blood cells being made by the body, or high rate of red blood cells being destroyed. The most common type of anemia is iron-deficiency anemia. If your blood is low in iron, it can't make hemoglobin. Typical causes of iron anemia are a diet low in iron, your body's inability to absorb iron, or blood loss. From what? Heavy periods in younger women, gastrointestinal bleeding, alcohol abuse that causes gastric ulcers, inflammatory or autoimmune diseases, and chronic infections are at the top of the list.

Because anemia literally starves your body of oxygen, anemia is a powerful enemy of nutritional support of any kind. Oxygen is very important for the body, but anemia deprives your red blood cells of much-needed oxygen. The basic functions of red blood cells are to maintain, regenerate, and heal the body. Without enough oxygen, they simply cannot operate adequately.

Whenever you work to manage a chronic health condition such as Hashimoto's, it is vital to test for anemia. Why? Because this could be the underlying reason you feel lousy. Anemia can be caused by a variety of factors, including B12 anemia (also known as pernicious anemia); which is an autoimmune B12 deficiency not uncommon in people with Hashimoto's. Some forms of anemia

50

don't respond to iron supplements, because the red blood cells in the body are breaking down. When this happens, supplementing will not increase iron levels and can make existing health problems much worse. Anemia can be a complex condition with many causes.

So how can you get the iron you need? **You will absorb 2 to 3 times more iron from animal sources than from plants.** Some of the best dietary sources are lean beef, turkey, chicken, lean pork, and fish. Some great plant sources are pinto, kidney beans, lentils, and dark green leafy vegetables, such as spinach.

The bottom line, ladies, is this: don't let your health be an unsolved mystery. Have your iron status checked. Anemia needs to be successfully addressed to overcome thyroid issues.

Check Blood Sugar Levels

When you were a good little girl, did you get treats? Comfort food was Oreo cookies and milk at the kitchen table with my mom. As an adult, for whatever emotion I was experiencing, or a girlfriend was experiencing, it was Starbucks mocha lattes, or festive cupcakes brought into the office to celebrate Monday. I was a sugar-holic, and believe me I know that sweets can seduce me in a heartbeat.

I believe sugar should be considered an illegal drug! It's sugar, not fat, that puts weight on, causes heart attacks, fills the mind with demons, robs you of minerals, rots your teeth, and causes inflammation, diabetes and cancer. It makes you feel high, like a new relationship, and then drops you flat like a bad man that just keeps you begging for more.

The U.S. Dietary guidelines have no limit for added sugar, and the FDA lists sugar as "generally regarded as safe (GRAS)." This lets the food industry add unlimited amounts of sugar or high fructose corn syrup to our food. It used to be that sugar was the only game in town to satisfy a sweet tooth. Then companies started pumping out chemical sweeteners like NutraSweet, Equal, Sweet and Low, saccharin and Splenda. "Artificial sweeteners are potent nerve toxins that never should have been approved as safe for consumption," said Dr. Ginger Southall of the Hippocrates Health Institute (Carr, 2011). Artificial sweeteners can damage your nervous system, causing seizures, depression, headaches, and unexplained visual problems. Many of your favorite foods have hidden artificial sweeteners, like Crystal light, flavored waters, condiments to include salad dressings, and even over the counter medicines like Alka-Seltzer! It is hard to limit sugar intake when processed foods such as breadcrumbs, applesauce, and cough syrups include hidden high fructose corn syrup. The US Dept. of Agriculture estimates that Americans eat an average of 150 lbs of sugar a year! That's a lot of cake, Girlfriend. It's not sexy, and it does not serve your beautiful body and brain.

Here are just a few facts to increase your understanding of what happens when you eat sugar. First, when glucose enters your bloodstream, the pancreas releases insulin. Insulin helps metabolize calories and regulates glucose levels by escorting it to cells to use as fuel. If the cell has all the fuel it needs, insulin carries the extra glucose to be stored as fat. This can turn into a downward cascade of falling dominoes if you eat too much sugar. Over time you can develop insulin resistance, which makes your body less effective at regulating blood sugar, burning fat for energy, or losing weight, and is a major cause of Diabetes, cancer, and autoimmune issues.

Everything we eat gets broken down to glucose eventually, even fats and proteins, because it is the fuel that feeds our cells. So how do we monitor our sugar intake? Voila, the Glycemic Index (GI). This is a measure of how quickly and how high a particular carbohydrate raises blood sugar. Since white sugar is all carbohydrate, it's designated as 100 on a scale of 0 to 100. Foods with a high GI value are usually highly refined simple carbs. As a rule of thumb, any foods with a ranking of 60 or lower are better for you. Examples are apples (38), black beans (30), strawberries (40). The GI Handbook by Barbara Ravage is a great resource.

Balanced blood sugar plays a huge role in managing hypothyroidism. Functional or optimal fasting blood glucose level ranges are 85 to 99. A fasting (no food or drink, except water, for 12 hours) blood sugar over 100 is considered insulin resistance, or pre-diabetes, and anything above 127 is diabetes.

A fasting blood glucose below 85 is considered hypoglycemia (low blood sugar) and a level above 99 is considered hyperglycemia (high blood sugar.) Both of these conditions are typically related to excess carbohydrates in the diet, and increase your risk of developing diabetes. Maintaining stable blood sugar is essential for your metabolism, energy, and hormones, and will help you regain your mojo. The best way to stabilize blood sugar?

There's no way around it, girlfriend, you've got to eat healthy foods with a low Glycemic Index.

The Role of Prolactin

Prolactin is a hormone made by your pituitary gland. It is best known for its role in lactation but also serves many other hormonal and metabolic roles. High levels of prolactin in the body suppress thyroid activity. How, you ask? The hormone progesterone and the neurotransmitter dopamine balance prolactin. When there is a progesterone or dopamine deficiency, levels of prolactin will increase, thus decreasing thyroid activity. This imbalance shows up on labs in the form of a low level of TSH (thyroid stimulating hormone), but perhaps not out of the lab reference range.

Prolactin also suppresses luteinizing hormone, which helps regulate the menstrual cycle and egg production, and excess prolactin can cause infertility. Sometimes high prolactin is caused by tumors called prolactinomas. The bottom line is that excess levels of prolactin, whether caused by a tumor or something else, can suppress your thyroid function, and suppressed thyroid function can cause chronic fatigue and pain.

Gluten Sensitivity

If your autoimmune issues were the subject of a noir mystery novel, do you know who the most notorious gangster would be? The mobster who has a hand in all the corruption and imbalance? Girlfriends, it would be gluten! Gluten is one of the biggest culprits for causing an autoimmune condition. Studies link Hashimoto's with gluten intolerance and celiac disease (Duntas, 2009), so it's especially important to avoid gluten if you have this disease. Gluten is most commonly found in wheat, rye, oats, barley, spelt, kamut, and triticale.

Have you noticed that gluten-free diets are all the rage these days? Some experts will tell you that this is just a fad. But the truth is more people are sensitive to gluten today than 75 years ago. **The reason so many people are now gluten-sensitive is that wheat has been engineered to be a much different protein than it was before 1940.** Before biotech companies began genetically modifying foods by inserting DNA from other organisms, farmers hybridized their crops in more natural ways. They chose the crops that presented the most desirable traits (such as higher yields, a better taste, or drought resistance) and bred them together to get one crop with as many desirable traits as possible -- kind of like breeding a pug and a beagle together to get an adorable puggle.

Today's wheat is shorter, browner, and higher yielding than it was a hundred years ago. These benefits came with a cost; the gluten proteins in wheat have changed, too. Our bodies were not made to eat this genetically hybridized wheat, and therefore the body considers it to be inflammatory. If you are sensitive to gluten and have an autoimmune condition, then when you eat anything that contains gluten – whether its cookies, a wheat roll, or pasta – your immune system attacks your body, the thyroid, joints, pancreas, or other tissue or organ.

There has yet to be a person with autoimmunity in my office who is not gluten-sensitive, and often sensitive to dairy, eggs, soy, yeast, and other foods as well. I know that cutting gluten or dairy or any other staple from your diet can be challenging. But if eating a cookie is the difference between dragging yourself out of bed, or dancing your way through your morning routine, isn't it worth the change? My mojo-touting body has been gluten free since 2007 and after those first few weeks, I've never looked back. If you truly want to feel better ThyroSisters, take control of your health and make the choice that works for you!

Vitamin D Deficiency

When you have an autoimmune disease, there are a lot of things to consider. It's like putting together a puzzle: if even one piece is missing, your health picture is incomplete. One of the most important pieces to achieving optimal health is making sure you're getting the nutrients your body needs. Vitamin D is an important nutrient, especially when it comes to healing Hashimoto's hypothyroidism, chronic fatigue, a lack of brain function, hormone imbalances, or any autoimmune condition. That's why it's so important to take therapeutic doses of vitamin D3 to support your immune system.

Vitamin D is a group of fat-soluble vitamins responsible for enhancing intestinal absorption of calcium, which is one of the bone's main building blocks. In humans, the most important compounds in this group are vitamin D3 (cholecalciferol) and vitamin D2 (ergocalciferol). When you get outside into the sunshine you get vitamins D and D2.

Modern diets often lack foods rich in vitamin D such as organ meats, lard, seafood, butter, and egg yolks. Autoimmune rates have skyrocketed during the past 20 years, while vitamin D levels have plummeted. Adequate vitamin D levels help to balance the immune system so it doesn't swing out of control, as it does in the presence of an autoimmune disease. In the modern diet, vitamin D can be found in fatty fish such as salmon, tuna or mackerel, and almost all US milk is fortified with 400iu of vitamin D per quart. Some breakfast cereals add vitamin D as well.

Many people, especially those suffering from diabetes, lupus, Hashimoto's, or fibromyalgia, need higher amounts of Vitamin D to maintain good health, even if tests show they have sufficient Vitamin D. This is due to a genetic issue that makes it difficult to absorb vitamin D.

It is possible to consume too much vitamin D, so do not take supplements without first having your blood levels tested, then you know how deficient you are and have a base line to check progress. Ask your doctor to order blood tests for Vitamin D,25-Hydroxycalciferol, the storage form, and Vitamin D, 1,25 Dihydroxy (Calcitriol), the active form. If your Vitamin D level is low, you need to take Vitamin D supplements. Eating plenty of fish oil and other foods rich in omega 3 fatty acids also helps when you have an autoimmune condition.

Now, putting together the puzzle pieces of your health may feel a bit overwhelming at this point. Like any puzzle, we're just beginning to pull out all the pieces to study them closely. Are you wondering how in the world you'll get from a pile of seemingly random pieces into a picture of mojo-filled health? Well, don't fret! I'm here to help you organize the pieces and plan your strategy. Just hang in there and we'll get that puzzle built. Besides, putting together a puzzle is more fun with a friend, right?

Adrenal Gland Stress

Earlier I talked about how, throughout our lives, stress can burn out our adrenal glands until they turn into dried up pieces of toast. But healthy adrenal glands, which secrete stress hormones such as cortisol, are vital for optimal health and the management of autoimmune diseases. Cortisol plays a large role in balancing the immune system by telling the body whether to go into "stress mode" and increase immunity efforts. **When the adrenal glands release cortisol, the cortisol is accompanied by cytokines, which are inflammatory messengers.**

High cortisol levels in the body reflect chronic inflammation, which leads to an eventual breakdown of the hormone system and the thyroid. Common causes of elevated cortisol and cytokines include chronic stress, post-traumatic stress disorder (PTSD), or hidden gut infections, such as parasites. Other causes of elevated cortisol levels include hypoglycemia, insulin resistance, and diabetes. Keeping blood sugar stable is an important factor in managing cortisol as well. Let's turn these burnt-up little pieces of toast into loaves of fluffy, sprouted grain that will help regulate cortisol levels for many years to come!

Understanding Leaky Gut

Have you heard the term leaky gut? Sounds pretty gross just from the name, doesn't it?

In leaky gut, a trigger substance (like parasites, or gluten or dairy if you're sensitive) damages the lining of the small intestines, opening up tight junctions that normally keep the intestinal wall impermeable. As a result, large molecules from food "leak" through the intestinal wall into the blood stream. The immune system reads these invaders the same as bacteria and viruses, as the enemy, and creates antibodies to destroy them. This response can set up a whole cascade of trouble to include rashes, respiratory tract and sinus problems, joint pain, brain fog, weight gain and fluid retention.

Gut function is extremely important when managing any type of autoimmune disorder. Leaky gut is a primary culprit to intestinal issues, although often there are no obvious symptoms. The intestinal tract becomes leaky due to chronic inflammation that breaks open or widens the normally tight junctions of the intestinal mucosa, causing a further cycle of inflammation. This in turn causes damage to the cells and the ability to digest fats, carbohydrates, or proteins effectively. This cascade of events happens because the small villi, or hairs, in the intestinal tract weaken and are unable to absorb nutrients. The "tight junctions" that hold the mucosal lining together break open, and the immune system launches an invasion against the toxins in the bloodstream, causing global inflammation.

Women often ask me, "How did this happen?" The studies suggest that leaky gut is partly due to chronic stress, even if you have "mal-adapted" to the stress, often your body has not. (Gareau MG, 2008), and also the negative impact of environmental toxins, unknown autoimmune, and food sensitivities (Pinton P, 237 (1)). What can you do about it? A lot! I will go into more detail about this; making critical lifestyle changes will make a huge difference in healing your gut.

You need to know if you have a leaky gut and if your digestive tract is functioning properly. Imagine that your picture of health contains one puzzle piece that touches nearly every other piece; it's edges reaching out like tentacles to touch not just digestion, but brain function, the immune system, hormone regulation, and cardiovascular health. Similar to the bacteria that aids in digestion, your gut is an integral part of your body's ecosystem. Throw it out of whack, and you will have problems you don't initially seem related to gut health, like proper thyroid function. A healthy gut also keeps you running with high energy, keeps the brain balanced and helps you absorb nutrients to keep your hormones balanced and well-functioning. That's a pretty important puzzle piece, isn't it?

Polycystic Ovarian Syndrome

Being a woman comes with some amazing life experiences. Our bodies can create life from a few strings of DNA and a uterus. Okay, so that's a bit of an oversimplification. But our feminine bodies can do some amazing things that men will never experience. The downside is that we may also experience health issues that are unique to our sex.

One of these issues is PCOS (Polycystic Ovarian Syndrome), where the ovaries become enlarged and many small cysts appear on them. PCOS is a health problem that can negatively affect a women's ability to have children, contribute to heart issues, and cause issues with the menstrual cycle. The cause is unknown. Experts speculate that factors such as genetics may play a role, but the main underlying problem is usually hormone imbalances. Women with PCOS make more testosterone from the ovaries than normal, which affects the development and release of eggs during ovulation.

Studies show that Polycystic Ovarian Syndrome (PCOS) can trigger Hashimoto's and other autoimmune diseases (Koeman, 2012). **PCOS is a common female hormone disorder, affecting almost 10 percent of menstruating women, and almost 30 percent of obese women.** It is a hormone imbalance characterized by menstrual irregularities, ovarian cysts, and high testosterone, and it is one of the most common causes of infertility.

PCOS symptoms include the inability to lose weight, hair loss, fatigue after meals, hormone imbalances, and sugar cravings. Blood sugar imbalances—primarily insulin resistance—are a main cause of PCOS.

Insulin resistance (pre-diabetes) is indicated by a fasting blood glucose level over 100, fatigue after meals, excess belly fat, and elevated triglycerides and cholesterol; especially if the triglycerides are higher than the cholesterol levels. This condition occurs when the body's cells become resistant to insulin, due primarily to eating a high carbohydrate diet. This leads to excess testosterone production, which in turn cascades into PCOS. As testosterone levels rise, the cells become further resistant to insulin.

Having insulin resistance also promotes inflammation and immune imbalances, which predispose a person to an autoimmune disease. Combine this chain of events with Hashimoto's disease, and you can see why treating PCOS is an important piece of the fatigue and hypothyroidism puzzle.

Got Hashimoto's? Take the Bull by the Horns

Now that we've looked at multiple puzzle pieces, it's time to start taking action. If you discover that your symptoms are the result of an underactive thyroid or other autoimmune disorder, this knowledge provides a great deal of the information you need to regain your mojo. It's now up to you to take your health care into your own hands! Start by working with a doctor who looks at the big picture, does thorough testing, and treats you appropriately based on the test results.

We are conditioned to believe that medical doctors know best, but simply ordering a TSH test, interpreting the results incorrectly, or writing a prescription for thyroid meds isn't fully diagnosing or treating someone with an underactive thyroid. With a disease as complex as Hashimoto's, or other chronic autoimmune conditions, you have to grab the bull by the horns and take charge of your body, and your life. Sometimes you may need to get a second or third opinion. Consider taking a more functional approach. And be your own health advocate, because it's your body and your life. If you know something just isn't right with your health, don't give up!

What is your life plan for the next 30 or 40 years? It's exhausting to go from doctor to doctor searching for answers that aren't forthcoming, or enduring the thinning patience of your family, but now is not the time to give up! After all, why are you reading this book if not to continue to fight for the return of your mojo?

No one else is ultimately responsible for your life and health, and no one knows your body as well as you do. If you've started to lose interest in caring for yourself, or are unsure what to do next, then all the more reason to create an action plan now, before the situation gets any worse. The key to getting your mojo back is to correctly identify the core cause of your symptoms. You need to get the appropriate tests done now, and a thorough workup to evaluate the cause of your symptoms. The best way to regain vibrancy in your life is with proper testing, treatment, and support.

If your current plan is to sit around and wait for your health problems to go away, or if you think nothing can be done, you are falling into a deep, dark well. Do your best to avoid this type of thinking by keeping in mind that it will not yield positive results. **Once you get properly tested and treated, you will regain your health and improve your sense of well-being.** Find a doctor who treats you as a whole person and uses functional, neurologic, and metabolic protocols. Life is short, very short, and ignorance is not bliss—ignorance is pain.

4 CLUES SUGGESTING
A THYROID AUTOIMMUNE DISEASE

1. **The presence of other autoimmune diseases.**

2. **Symptoms that come and go.**

3. **Supplement solutions aren't working.**

4. **Significant symptoms began after a major stressor.**

- Get your vitamin D levels tested, and if needed begin vitamin D supplementation until blood levels return to normal, and your symptoms improve.

- Monitor your essential fatty acid intake and take a high-quality fish oil.

- Test, don't guess! I highly recommend the gluten panel from Cyrex Labs (www.cyrexlabs.com) because it tests for the many different components of gluten that people react to, not just alpha gliadin.

CHAPTER 4
THE UNBALANCED PUZZLE PIECE:
Is Your Body Hormonally Happy?

" For beautiful eyes, look for good in others. For beautiful lips, speak only words of kindness. And for poise, walk with the knowledge you are never alone. **"**

Audrey Hepburn

Doctors had diagnosed Alaina, age 45, with

hypothyroidism ten years ago. Although she was taking thyroid hormone medication, her symptoms of fatigue, depression, weight gain, and brain fog worsened over the years. To make it through her days as a flight attendant, she drank caffeinated tea and energy drinks, even though they gave her migraines. She spent her days off in bed sleeping. Her memory was slipping, and she found it increasingly difficult to concentrate.

Alaina happened to be working during a flight I was on when she saw some nutritional supplements in my bag and asked me about them. I talked to her about hypothyroidism and how to stay hormonally healthy during the menopausal years. A month later Alaina came to see me as a patient. The first thing I did was a panel of lab tests to verify that Hashimoto's disease was responsible for her low energy, depression, and weight gain. Alaina's doctor wanted to put her on antidepressant medication. I said, "You don't need antidepressants. Let's go after the autoimmune disease instead."

I approached improving Alaina's condition in several different ways. The first was improving her diet. Alaina cried for two days after I told her to give up gluten. She had just lost her mother, and all her favorite comfort foods contained gluten. Nevertheless, she followed my advice and was amazed when she felt significantly better after three days of being on a gluten-free diet.

"Dr. Labbe told me I would feel like a million bucks, and I was like, 'Yeah, right,'" says Alaina. "She was right! Going gluten-free is a drastic diet, but I was shocked how quickly I started to feel better."

A gluten-free diet is necessary to quench an autoimmune reaction, but other steps are vital as well. They include taking Vitamin D and Omega 3 supplements and loading up on glutathione, the most powerful antioxidant. The next step in helping Alaina was to determine how best to balance her immune system. When someone has an autoimmune disease, such as Hashimoto's, this is a strong indication that the immune system is wildly out of balance. I used lab tests and other evaluations to determine the specific nature of Alaina's nutritional and hormonal imbalances. I checked for adrenal fatigue through a saliva test that measures cortisol and compares the measurement from morning, noon, and night. Anemia was a concern due to her severe fatigue. We checked for iron anemia as well as B12/folic acid anemia. TPO and TGB antibodies were checked for thyroid auto immune issues, as well as free T3, T4 and T7 (described in depth in chapter 3). Progesterone, estrogen, and testosterone were checked through a saliva test and a urine test for neurotransmitters (including serotonin, gabba, and dopamine was performed.)

The test results would provide answers as to why Alaina wasn't sleeping and kept fighting the "blues." She was excited and hopeful to know these tests are available! Just knowing these tests exist can empower you to talk with your health practitioner to run the tests in order to get to the root cause of your symptoms and loss of mojo. Many of my clients never knew they could find out what their serotonin levels are, or that there is an important circadian rhythm to cortisol.

Alaina and I agreed on a plan that included supplements to help support healthy hormone levels, such as a special extract of Siberian rhubarb, ERr 731, that's been shown in clinical studies to significantly reduce hot flashes. Can you imagine? I have experienced tremendous results with this supplement in reducing hot flashes. This extract of rhubarb doesn't contain estrogens, and has proven to be a safe alternative treatment for hot flashes. Researchers are not clear how ERr 731 performs it's actions in the body. I have found that 4 milligrams have significantly reduced the frequency and severity of hot flashes in menopausal women (Heger, 2006). Vitamin D3 with K2 helped balance Alaina's hormones and support calcium levels. To improve sleep she started taking 800 mg of magnesium, and a non habit-forming supplement that contains 4-amino-3phenylbutyric acid melatonin, and 5-hydroxytryptophan (from Griffonia simplicifolia seed extract). Finally, to help Alaina's thyroid levels, I recommended a product with a high-quality bovine thyroid glandular, including amino acids, fatty acids, and a rich mix of herbal and nutritional compounds to support the thyroid gland, thyroid hormone physiology, and thyroid hormone receptor binding, as well as to promote T3 and T4 production.

Dog Tired to the Bone

Now if you were to raise your hand and state your biggest concern, I bet it would be fatigue! I see many hands out there. To help increase her energy levels, Alaina began taking a powdered formula drink that reduces fatigue by restoring ATP in the mitochondria. Mitochondria are tiny organelles found in every cell in the body, and are responsible for creating more than 90% of cellular energy, sustaining life, and supporting growth of the cells. ATP (adenosine triphosphate) is your best friend when it comes to energy. It is a high-energy molecule that, when broken down into ADP, creates energy that drives many important reactions in the cell.

In the fight against fatigue, it's important that you understand how the importance of the ThyroSister ATP and how she likes to roll. If you take care of ATP, she'll help you keep fatigue from frying your life.

There are several compounds that help maximize ATP's energy productivity:

D-Ribose is a naturally occurring sugar that supports the production and recycling of ATP, helping to increase energy formation in stressed tissues.

DMG (dimethylglycine) is a powerhouse that helps the body overcome various forms of stress, aging, poor oxygen supply, and free radical damage. It contributes methyl groups to help keep ATP levels (your new best friend) high.

CoQ10 is an anti-oxidant vital to the production of ATP; it improves the heart's pumping ability and tone, and protects the heart from free radical damage. CoQ10 levels decline after age 40 (Langsjoen PH, 2003), so it's important to supplement.

Acetyl-L-Carnitine is a derivative of the amino acid carnitine. It supports heart function by transporting fatty acids from the blood to the mitochondria of the heart cells and converting them into your friend ATP. Your big, beautiful heart needs a constant supply of ATP to keep beating regularly, and Acetyl-L Carnitine helps make that happen.

Malic Acid, a magnificent player, is involved in energy production in muscle cells, along with protease and bromelain (proteolytic enzymes that decrease muscle soreness following exercise or other activities). Together they nourish muscles, nerves, and even help with glucose metabolism, which helps with weight management.

You too can soon enjoy a renewed sense of energy, freedom, and vitality. I know you feel like you've been tired for so long that there is no way you can re-boot. What I'm recommending is supplementing your energy, not a part-time quick energy boost that fizzles out and leaves you feeling more tired than before. I'm recommending a change in lifestyle, embracing a new way to age with grace, and no longer having to fret about fatigue, weight, brain fog, indigestion, insomnia, or other unpleasant symptoms often associated with menopause. This is a new, fabulous season that will set the stage for the rest of your long, robust life!

How Stressed Are You?

It is a constant refrain: we're too stressed out. But how stressed are we really? There are two types of stress, physiological stress (the stress placed on your body when not all of your systems are working properly) and everyday stress (emotional stress caused by things like long days at work, getting dinner on the table before the kids have to start homework, and not having time to relax), and the two can sometimes seem totally unrelated. For instance, you may feel like, overall you have a mellow personality, but your stress hormone levels could be off the charts due to chronic inflammation or other imbalances in your body.

Your adrenal glands are two small glands that sit atop each kidney. They secrete stress hormones, including cortisol, that help you cope with stress and play an important role in many bodily systems. When you suffer from chronic stress your cortisol levels can get too high, or your adrenal function can become so overworked that the body releases too little cortisol, a condition known as adrenal fatigue.

The good news is that we don't have to guess. We can test how well or poorly the adrenal glands are functioning with a simple yet powerful home test kit you can order from my website www.ThyroSisters.com. It's called an *Adrenal Saliva Test.* There are four vials in the kit labeled Morning, Afternoon, Night, and Midnight. You simply spit (yes, Sweet Thing you can spit) in these vials during one day, no fasting, and send the specimens (the saliva) off to the lab in the pre-labeled secure container.

This test will show whether your cortisol (the stress hormone) is too high or too low and provides insight into which stage of adrenal fatigue your body is in. There are seven stages of adrenal function, one being the best, seven being total adrenal fatigue. Taking a saliva reading throughout the day provides a more accurate diagnostic than just drawing blood. The blood draw tells us "at that moment in time" what your cortisol level is, but your levels change throughout the day due to circadian rhythms, your activity level, etc.

Cortisol plays a huge part in why you are tired, can't lose weight, and can't sleep. Both adrenal fatigue and excess adrenal hormones can throw off your mojo, big-time. Either situation will make a messy mixture of your hormones and creates a rough menopausal transition, and there is a lot we can do to turn this around, once we know the lay of the land from doing the right tests.

Symptoms of adrenal fatigue are:
- Fatigue
- Slow to get moving in the morning
- Energy crash in the afternoon
- Craving sweets, caffeine, or nicotine
- Unstable behavior/moodiness
- Shaky, lightheaded, or irritable when meals are delayed
- Inability to stay asleep
- Dizziness when moving from sitting to standing

Symptoms of excess adrenal hormones are:
• Excess belly fat
• Insulin resistance
• Insomnia
• Not feeling rested in the morning
• Increased growth of facial hair
• Polycystic Ovarian Syndrome (PCOS)

You can measure how much stress your body is experiencing through the Adrenal Saliva Test. Measuring stress levels not only uncovers the reasons for feeling chronically cruddy, but can also chart the level of improvement achieved while following a health protocol. There are many saliva tests available to evaluate adrenal function; the one I use and recommend is the Adrenal Stress Index test available through Metametrix Laboratory (www.metametrix.com), or Diagnos-Techs (www.diagnostechs.com).

These tests measure cortisol levels (a master stress hormone impacting many bodily systems), dehydroepiandrosterone (DHEA is a precursor to testosterone and estrogens), and 17-hydroxyprogesterone (a precursor to cortisol.) The lab analysis of the saliva reveals whether your stress hormone levels are too high or too low, provides information about your circadian rhythms (sleep-wake cycle), and shows whether your symptoms are from adrenal fatigue or overactive adrenal function. The saliva test results also show whether you suffer from the "alarm reaction" of overactive adrenal glands, or from exhaustion of the adrenal glands. Contrary to popular belief, one does not necessarily slide gradually from alarm reaction to adrenal fatigue. Adrenal function can jump around between phases, or stay in one phase for years.

In addition, the adrenal saliva test measures the total SIgA (secretory antibodies) that are made by the immune system, and are a kind of master cell. Think of this as a blank key the immune system uses to make more immune cells that specialize in different functions. We want healthy levels of SIgA, so the immune system has plenty of raw materials to work with when fighting infections and invaders. Your SIgA level shows the impact that stress has taken on your immune system. When it's low the immune system is weakened, making you more susceptible to food intolerances, infections, and other "assaults."

The Importance of Circadian Rhythms

The adrenal glands secrete cortisol at different levels throughout the day. Measuring the level of stress hormones at different times of the day reveals your individual circadian rhythm, or sleep-wake cycle. In a healthy body cortisol secretion is highest in the morning and lowest at night, so you feel alert when you wake up, and tired before going to bed.

How many people do you know who can't fall asleep at night, barely crawl out of bed in the morning, or bolt awake in the middle of the night? Perhaps you are one of them. **Many people have a reversed circadian rhythm that causes fatigue in the morning and insomnia at night.** Or instead of declining gradually throughout the day, their cortisol levels drop suddenly in the afternoon, causing an afternoon crash that sends them staggering to Starbucks for a caffeine and sugar fix (caffeine, by the way, is not good for ailing adrenal glands). Overstressed adrenal glands can also fluctuate wildly, sending cortisol levels surging and dropping throughout the day, creating dramatic highs and lows in energy.

When the Body Attacks the Adrenal Glands

Another important step in understanding the status of your adrenal glands is to test whether you are having an autoimmune reaction in which the immune system erroneously attacks and destroys the tissue it was designed to protect. I've already discussed the problems caused by autoimmunity, so just keep in mind that if you suffer from persistent and chronic low levels of cortisol, or experience adrenal fatigue, an autoimmune reaction related to the adrenal glands is worth investigating.

Poor adrenal function is always secondary to something else, but if you've ruled out other possibilities, an autoimmune reaction could be to blame. Fortunately, a blood-panel that tests for antibodies to 21-hydroxylase (an antigen associated with adrenal autoimmunity or insufficiency) will determine whether the immune system is attacking and destroying the adrenal glands, thus causing adrenal insufficiency.

If the results are positive, then you will need to effectively manage your immune system; in addition to supporting your adrenal health. If this turns out to be your health challenge, think of this information as a gift. You'll finally know the root cause, or causes, of the symptoms that are wreaking havoc with your health. Now you have a much clearer process for healing and getting back your mojo.

COMMON SYMPTOMS OF HORMONAL IMBALANCE:

- Poor bone health
- Difficulty getting a good night's sleep
- Dry, saggy skin
- Thyroid disorder
- Poor memory
- Migraine headaches
- Low sex drive
- Worry and anxiety
- Joint pain

Why Adrenal Hormones Are Important

Whether test results indicate that your adrenal glands are tired and worn out, or supercharged and overactive, the resulting hormonal imbalance leads to a number of chronic health problems. Do any of these problems sound familiar?

• *Poor Bone Health*

Abnormal circadian rhythms compromise tissue healing and repair, increase muscle and joint breakdown, and can cause chronic joint pain. In fact, for middle-aged women, stress is the enemy of bone health as cortisol levels determine how well we build and maintain healthy bones. Therefore chronically high levels make us more prone to bone loss and osteoporosis.

• *Sleep Disturbances*

Cortisol imbalances also disrupt the quality of our sleep. Too much cortisol secretion at night compromises your ability to enter into regenerative sleep cycles. Chronic lack of regenerative sleep zaps your mojo, reduces your overall vitality, and can even induce depression.

Adrenal fatigue, with its irregular output of cortisol can also sabotage your sleep. You would think being tired all the time would be great for sleep. And for many it is, although some with low levels need 10 or more hours of sleep to function. But the body needs melatonin (the sleep hormone) to sleep well, and sufficient cortisol is needed to manufacture this hormone. When cortisol levels are low, melatonin levels drop and sleep quality is poor.

Cortisol also triggers the processes that keep the brain supplied with energy during a long night with no food. However, when cortisol is too low, the fight-or-flight hormones will kick in to compensate. When they gear up to fuel an energy-starved brain around 2 or 3 AM, this will shock you awake. Anxiety and worry are often side effects of this wake-up call.

• *Aging Skin*
Aging skin is no joke. Maybe if you're saintly you don't care about the sags, the dry skin, the droops and lines, but the hundreds of billions of dollars spent on anti-aging skin products and treatments every year suggests that most of us care very much.

So hear this, chronic stress ages your skin…fast. If you aren't concerned about what adrenal malfunction does to your bones, brain, or hormones, know that the negative effects will eventually show up on your pretty face. Human skin regenerates mostly during the night. When adrenal function is imbalanced and cortisol is high and disrupting sleep, less skin regeneration takes place.

Have you seen photos of U.S. presidents before and after their presidency? If you toss and turn at night and feel as though the weight of the Western World is on your shoulders, you may develop baggy eyes and saggy skin in just a few years if you don't effectively manage your stress levels. Healthy adrenal function is essential for optimum skin health.

• *Poor Thyroid Health*
Symptoms of an underactive thyroid, such as fatigue or low body temperature, are often due to adrenal imbalance. **Chronic stress can also cause the pituitary gland (which directs hormone function) to become fatigued.** This happens because fluctuations in the thyroid gland influence neurological signaling going on from your adrenal glands to the hypothalamus, where the pituitary gland is located.

One consequence is that your body doesn't produce enough thyroid hormone. When this happens, symptoms that you wouldn't normally associate with the thyroid start to plague your life: brain fog, forgetfulness, difficulties losing weight even when doing everything "right," feeling tired after you eat, and sleeping poorly.

Improving Hormone Health

The bottom line is this: for a woman grappling with hormonal upheavals, chronic stress can make a bad situation even worse. If you suffer from constant stress, lack of vitality, or muscle and joint pain; if you've been told you have hypoglycemia or insulin resistance; or if you experience migraine headaches, osteoporosis, sleep disturbances, poor memory, or low sex drive, finding out more about the health of your adrenal glands is essential.

The easiest way to do so is to take the saliva adrenal test; the results will provide the 'lay of the land' when it comes to your adrenal glands so you can better understand the root problem causing these issues. Then they can be corrected. Ahhhh yes, there is such a thing as an abundant, vibrant, sexy midlife!

I take several different approaches in providing adrenal support to my patients, depending on whether someone suffers from too much cortisol, adrenal fatigue, or an imbalanced circadian rhythm.

• **Adrenal adaptogens:** Whether dealing with too much or too little cortisol, adrenal adaptogen herbs are a group of herbal compounds used to improve the adrenal glands, and how you respond to stress and resist fatigue. They help to buffer stress, regulate circadian rhythm function in the brain, and improve mental function. Adaptogens work a little like your air conditioner when it is on "auto." When the sensors sense the room is too hot, it cools down the room; when the sensors read too cool, it turns on the heat and warms the room. Adaptogens help regulate cortisol levels and can relax you without making you tired, and boost your energy without making you jittery like coffee and sugar! They have been used since biblical times, and have been used in Indian Ayurvedic medicine for centuries. I use a combination of herbs and amino acids that include Panax ginseng, ashwagandha, holy basil, rhodiola, and eleuthero.

• **Phosphatidylserine (PS):** When the area of the brain responsible for learning and memory is ravaged by stress, causing high levels of cortisol, PS protects the hippocampus and lowers high cortisol levels. How does this work? Cortisol is released during any type of physical, mental, or emotional stress; it helps you during extreme stress. You probably have heard of the fight or flight response; this is created by cortisol, which is activated in amounts to help your body store fat (a source of fuel) and allow the body to use muscle as fuel. PS acts as a cortisol-blunting supplement in response to out-of-range cortisol. PS is difficult to obtain in an oral form, so I use a liposomal skin cream that delivers PS through the skin. Many women love its calming effect, which also helps to improve sleep.

• **For low cortisol:** For clients with adrenal fatigue and general low energy I recommend a liposomal skin cream that contains Glycyrrhiza glabra (made from licorice), which extends the life of cortisol and improves overall energy. I also use SAMe, 5-MTHF and Methylcobalamin; all support the synthesis of norepinephrine, dopamine, and serotonin in the brain.

• **For high cortisol:** In treating elevated cortisol levels, in addition to supplementing with phosphatidylserine, I recommend a formula made with Banaba leaf extract that reduces the production of cortisol. Formulas with glycine and taurine have additional calming support. Taurine is an amino acid that increases glycine and GABA to calm the brain, and protects the brain by reducing the harmful effects of excess glutamate (glutamate is the principal excitatory neurotransmitter in the brain).

Here's an update on Alaina's progress. Encouraged by the significant improvements she experienced from eliminating gluten from her diet, she followed my other recommendations, taking amino acids (L-lysine, N-acetyl L-cysteine, taurine, glycine and L-glutamine) to support her body's detoxification reactions, and also specific antioxidants, herbal extracts, and digestive enzymes. A big part of what helped Alaina was the addition of glutathione, a powerful antioxidant and detoxifier.

Her migraines diminished, and her high blood pressure returned to normal. The fatigue and depression she had been struggling with went away completely.

Though Alaina had been taking the same dose of thyroid medication for ten years, she found she needed to lower her dose after just one month on this program!

"Since turning my health around I have been able to work a lot of overtime," says Alaina. "At the end of a ten-hour work day my coworkers are exhausted, and I'm like the Energizer Bunny, ready to keep going."

Scientifically evaluating and improving the health of your adrenal glands can make a huge difference in how you feel and function. In Part Two of this book, I will share more tips and recommendations about ways to improve hormonal balance that will keep you and your hormones happy!

Secrets Whispered to a ThyroSister

To complete the Adrenal Stress Index test, you fill each of the four vials with saliva four times a day: First thing in the morning, during the day, in the late afternoon, and just before going to bed at night.

- Visit www.ThyroSisters.com/adrenalstressindex for more information on healing and assessing your adrenal health.

- If you suffer from symptoms of hormonal imbalance, get the Adrenal Stress Index saliva test kit from Diagnos-Techs (www.diagnostechs.com) or Metametrix Laboratory (www.metametrix.com)

- Let us help you correctly interpret the saliva test results to define whether you have adrenal fatigue, and if so what stage of exhaustion you have. With this information our highly trained team will recommend the appropriate adrenal support products for your situation.

- If you are suffering from low cortisol, or adrenal fatigue, you need to avoid refined sugar, alcohol, and caffeine as they further stress the immune system. Artificial additives such as aspartame or MSG are also very stressful to the adrenal glands.

- Check with your health practitioner about the advantages of taking natural ERr 731, extract of rhubarb, for hot flashes. You want to sizzle, but not because of hot flashes dear friends!

- Have your autoimmune antibodies checked against your adrenal glands. See if an antigen associated with adrenal autoimmune insufficiency, 21-hydroxylase, is contributing to your fatigue. (Cyrex Labs, Array 5)

- DMG, Acetyl-L-Carnitine, Malic Acid, and Liposomal Glutathione are all muscle men, power players, kicking sand in the face of fatigue!

CHAPTER 5
THE RED-EYED PUZZLE PIECE:
Do You Sleep Well at Night?

 The best cure for insomnia is to get a lot of sleep."

W.C. Fields

You know the problem with sleep, you're exhausted and looking forward to collapsing into bed at the end of the day, but as soon as your head hits the pillow, newfound energy courses through your body and your mind won't stop churning. Or perhaps you fall asleep quickly, but then bolt awake around 3 AM, with your mind alert and feeling worried or anxious

Lack of sleep, or poor quality sleep, have become a fact of life for more than 60 percent of Americans, fueling a $2 billion sleep-medication industry (Peterson, 2011). Many people use stimulants, such as coffee, energy drinks, and cigarettes to feel productive at work and fuel their activities during the day. Then they take medication to sleep at night, a pattern that makes sleep problems even worse. Furthermore, sleep deprivation increases the risk for developing health disorders such as Alzheimer's disease, obesity, depression, and heart disease. Not getting enough sleep, night after night, also speeds up the aging process. Clearly, not sleeping well at night is mojo-depleting, taking a significant toll on the mind and body.

Prescription sleeping pills are not the solution to the problem of sleeping poorly. While taking these medications may knock you out at night, their use frequently comes with troubling side effects, and can create more problems than they cure. The main problem with the treatments most doctors prescribe for insomnia is they don't address the root cause of the problem, but focus only on the symptom of not sleeping. When the medications to induce sleep stop working, which they will because the brain habituates to all stimuli, you often realize that they simply covered up the problem for a short time and did nothing to fix what's causing your insomnia in the first place.

Some doctors prescribe the newest medications on the market, some recommend antidepressants, and some even prescribe anti-seizure medications. All of these medications have side effects, and some are habit-forming. Insomnia is your body's way of telling you there is something wrong. If you take pills so you can sleep at night, and take more pills to get through the day, then you're making the problem worse by sabotaging your body's efforts to keep you balanced and healthy. Your body is trying to tell you something is wrong, but you're taking the batteries out of the fire alarm instead of looking for and putting out the fire!

If your doctor is treating you by covering up insomnia with medication, this is not solving the problem, or problems, that are at the core of not being able to sleep. Since none of the treatments your doctor is providing are meant to correct the insomnia, logic says your condition will continue to worsen. If you're like most of the long-term insomniacs I've helped, your life has become much less than it could be due to problems related to sleep deprivation, including feeling tired all the time.

A good night's rest, however, can do so much for your mojo. Sleep replenishes the body, heals injuries, backs up memories, and flushes out the mind. Even small interruptions in this process can lead to big issues; like a buggy computer with a full hard drive. If you don't do a disc cleanup on your computer every so often, it will eventually crash -- and so will your body if you don't sleep well.

So what are your options in addressing the factors that rob you of sleep? First of all, you need to figure out what is keeping you awake. The following are common causes of insomnia and ways to address them to get the "shut eye" you long for and deserve.

WHAT'S KEEPING YOU AWAKE?

- Eating excessive carbohydrates
- Imbalanced levels of brain chemicals
- Leaky gut
- Unidentified food sensitivities
- Hormones that are out of whack

Blood-Sugar Issues

The majority of sleep issues stem from diet related blood-sugar imbalances. Americans eat vastly more sweet and starchy foods – bread, pasta, rice, potatoes, pastry, dessert, sweetened coffee, and soda – than the human body was designed to handle --often more than twice a healthy amount (Jameson, 2010). This kind of diet usually leads to insulin resistance (from high blood sugar) or reactive hypoglycemia (from high insulin), both of which contribute to sleep disorders, and then not wanting to look at yourself in the mirror in the morning!

People who develop insulin resistance usually have high levels of adrenal stress hormones as well, as discussed in the previous chapter. Symptoms of adrenal stress hormones typically include difficulty falling asleep at night, or routinely waking up feeling as if you haven't slept at all. People with low blood sugar issues are also often bolting awake at 3 AM because their blood sugar drops during the night, triggering the production of stress hormones, which raises blood sugar and increases feelings of anxiety.

Eating a little protein, such as a handful of raw almonds, may help you successfully fall back to sleep. Also, in many cases eating a lower carbohydrate diet can significantly improve your sleep. I don't have hard and fast rules regarding how many grams of carbohydrates to eat, because carbohydrate needs vary from one person to another, but in most cases you should strive for less than 150 grams a day, the equivalent of five potatoes or two cups of pasta.

Imbalanced Brain Chemicals

The neurons in our brain use chemicals called neurotransmitters to communicate with one another. Sometimes this communication gets confused, causing numerous breakdowns in the body, including sleep disturbances, memory loss, weight gain, headaches, and low libido. What causes low neurotransmitters? They can be negatively affected by low-grade viral or bacterial infections, blood sugar imbalances, chronic stress, poor nutrition, toxic exposures, or genetics.

Maybe you have heard the adage; "early to bed, early to rise makes a ThyroSister healthy, wealthy, and wise!" Turns out that as far as great sleep is concerned, this is very true. Melatonin (the sleep hormone) naturally peaks between 9:00 PM and midnight. If you do not go to bed until midnight you have missed the opportunity to take advantage of melatonin as a natural sleep aid. If you go to bed closer to 9:00 PM you receive three hours of natural melatonin to help ease you into a restful slumber.

Women also need plenty of serotonin, or 5-hydroxytryptamine, a monoamine neurotransmitter. Biochemically derived from tryptophan, serotonin is primarily found in the gastrointestinal tract, yet another reason why you need your tummy to be intact, and not leaking. It's also found in blood platelets and the central nervous system (CNS). In the CNS, serotonin helps regulate mood, appetite, learning, memory, and of course, sleep.

Serotonin helps drive melatonin into performing its proper biochemical actions, which explains why a serotonin deficiency causes some degree of poor sleep for as many as 90 percent of Americans (Labbe, 2012). Boosting serotonin production with the amino acid L-tryptophan has proven effective for many people. I also like to round out L-tryptophan with L-lysine, which accelerates the production of the neurotransmitters serotonin and GABA in your brain. The natural function of GABA (Gamma-Amino Butyric Acid) is to inhibit (calm down) the activity of the neurons, another name for nerve cells. Some researchers believe that one of the purposes that GABA serves is to control the fear or anxiety experienced when neurons are overexcited. GABA helps calm and relax us, and a deficiency of GABA can be a reason why some people have anxiety disorders or panic attacks.

Impaired Gut Health

Believe it or not, bad bacteria in your gut can negatively affect your sleep! Under normal conditions the gut has ample beneficial bacteria to aid in digestion and many other functions. Unfortunately poor diet, stress, and other challenges can tip the balance so that the gut becomes infected with an overgrowth of harmful bacteria and fungi. Gross, right? And it won't be a delicious portabella mushroom growing in your stomach, either. The resulting infections from these overgrowths produce chemicals that aggravate the immune and nervous systems and trigger the release of the stress hormone cortisol. High levels of cortisol will interfere with your ability to fall asleep, or stay asleep.

Fortunately, stool and saliva tests will identify the type of gut infection you may have and indicate how it is negatively affecting your stress hormone levels. As always, it's important to test and not guess! There is a saliva/urine test kit (see www.ThyroSisters.com) that provides extraordinary information about the status of your cortisol, progesterone, estrogen, testosterone, and the neurotransmitters, serotonin, GABA, and dopamine. Armed with the results of these tests, I use a combination of botanical compounds and dietary approaches to restore health to the gut. Not only does addressing gut issues alleviate digestive problems, it also calms inflammation and reduces cortisol levels so that you sleep well throughout the night.

Sensitivities to Food

Perhaps surprisingly, another factor that can raise stress hormones and rob you of much-needed sleep is food sensitivities and food allergies. You may not realize that gluten, dairy, eggs, or other foods are triggering an immune response in your body. Food sensitivities increase the production of stress hormones and provoke inflammation, creating an environment in the gut that fosters bacterial and fungal infections.

Adopting an anti-inflammatory diet and gut-healing protocol paves the way to sweet slumber by reducing inflammation and the overproduction of stress hormones. After following this diet for a few weeks to a few months, depending on the severity of your inflammation, you might find that you can slowly reintroduce some of these foods back into your diet.

How Hormones Affect Your Sweet Slumber

One of the most common complaints from women going through perimenopause and menopause is the decreasing quality of their sleep. One reason is that the female brain depends on estrogen for healthy functioning, including keeping anxiety at bay, staying calm, and getting a good night's sleep. As a woman transitions through menopause, her ovaries gradually decrease production of estrogen and progesterone, which are sleep enhancing hormones.

When estrogen declines, so does serotonin activity, and sleep and mood problems are often the result. Also, waning estrogen may make you more sensitive to environmental stressors; for example you may be more sensitive to a dog barking, or a small amount of light coming from the streetlight outside the bedroom. You may also experience a hot flash, which is a surge of adrenaline, waking you up from a deep slumber and bathing you in sweat, and then taking a little time to get back to sleep.

Progesterone is known as the calming hormone and can powerfully influence sleep. Progesterone helps stimulate the release of GABA (gamma amino butyric acid), which helps induce sleep, calmness and well-being due to its natural "valium-like" effect. Because progesterone levels are negatively impacted by stress, progesterone deficiency is very common. Progesterone can also dip quite low during menopause, creating too much estrogen in relationship to progesterone, a situation called estrogen dominance.

Both your estrogen and progesterone levels may also be low. I recommend the adrenal-stress saliva test (introduced in the previous chapter) to my sleepless clients. It will show us the "lay of the land" in terms of current hormone levels, so you can lay your pretty head down and soon drift into restorative slumber. First, exhaust all the steps suggested to restore gut health and adrenal function. If doing so still does not boost your estrogen and progesterone levels, I might suggest using bioidentical hormone replacement (discussed at the beginning of this book) for a brief period of time for the hormonally imbalanced, sleep-deprived woman.

Are You Seeking a Sleep Supplement?

Certain supplements can improve sleep; many of them work by helping to calm the activity of the brain. The calming herbs include valerian, hops, passionflower, and chamomile. L-theanine is an amino acid that boosts the neurotransmitter GABA and calms the brain, it's found in green tea and is known for its ability to help with relaxation and focus.

GABA is technically an amino acid. It is produced in the brain from Glutamate (another amino acid and neurotransmitter) as well as vitamin B6. GABA is the chief inhibitory neurotransmitter, meaning it prevents over-excitement of your neurons from external stimuli. Low levels of this transmitter are linked to irregular sleep patterns, depression, anxiety, and overreaction to stress. GABA also increases the level of alpha waves in the brain, making you feel calm, focused, and in the zone.

Additional supplements that have proven wonderful for sleeping are 5-HTP and magnesium. Some people titrate up slowly on magnesium to 800 mg before bed. One product I recommend that has performed incredibly well for inducing restorative sleep includes the ingredients taurine and 4-amino-3-phenybutyric acid. Check out **http://www.ThyroSisters.com** for more information, including where you can get it.

Resolve today not to lie awake late at night anymore, wondering why you can't sleep; it's time to find answers that really work. Time is limited, and you have things to do, places to go, people to meet. If you have been struggling for over three months with sleep issues, this has become a chronic condition and is taking a toll on all aspects of your life. Find the cause of your sleep deprivation through testing and not guessing. Identify the causes through urine lab testing and questionnaires about your specific symptoms designed to get to the core cause of your sleepless nights. ThyroSisters, there are numerous solutions to your sleep problems.

Now that you understand the factors that have sapped your mojo over the years, you're in a position to create an effective plan for getting your health back and keeping it! In the process of exploring the common culprits that mooch mojo in midlife we've narrowed down the possibilities, identified your most troubling symptoms, defined the tests that provide clarity, and the supplements that offer solutions.

Now we will further explore the empowering lifestyle choices that are available to you, in addition to defining what you need from your health professional. ThyroSisters, continue with me on this healing journey – there are much brighter days ahead!

Secrets Whispered to a ThyroSister

More Tips for a Good Night's Sleep

- Set your alarm clock for an hour **before** you go to bed. Use this as a reminder to start winding down from your day. Turn off all the electronics; take a warm shower/bath, meditate, pray, or recall all the blessings of the day.
- Keep your bedroom as dark as possible for sleep, covering up all of the lights coming from electronic devices, even the LED light on the alarm clock, or wearing an eye mask.
- If you need to get up during the night, don't turn on the lights. This really wakes up the brain, making it difficult to go back to sleep. Memorize your way from your bed to the bathroom sweet girlfriend; so you return to sleep quickly.

- Visit www.ThyroSisters.com to learn more about the saliva test that will provide information about your circadian rhythms. *Is your cortisol too high at night? Is your progesterone too low? Is your insulin too low, or too high?* With this test you'll find out.

- Repair leaky gut if this is an issue for you. It will make a significant difference in your health, and decrease inflammation. Working on gut repair is paramount to taming autoimmunity and helping you feel better.

- The sleep hormone, melatonin, normally surges between 9:00 pm and midnight. So the later you go to bed, the more you increase your chances of missing the natural melatonin cycle.

- Include a non-addictive, no hangover supplement to promote the onset and quality of sleep. The ingredients I've seen work best are a GABA derivative, 4-amino-3-phenylbutyric acid, 5-HTP, and melatonin. All help promote restorative sleep by calming neurotransmitters and hormones.

- Magnesium is a powerful mineral that affects over 350 biochemical pathways in our body, and it's a huge player in helping you sleep. Slowly increase to taking as much as 800 milligrams before bedtime.

PART TWO:
Putting The Pieces Together:
How To Get Your Mojo Back,
And How To Keep It!

In part one we explored the often overlooked reasons for feeling fuzzy, funky, frazzled, or fatigued, and discussed solutions to diagnose and treat mojo-depleting issues, to include specialized blood testing, supplements, healing nutrition, and lifestyle changes. This second section explores each piece of the health puzzle in more depth and detail, explaining even more empowering steps that will bring you the solutions you seek and describing ways to re-build yourself to regain vibrant health.

CHAPTER 6
BUILDING FROM THE INSIDE OUT:
Healthy Gut

> **"** The best day of your life is the one on which you decide your life is your own. No apologies or excuses. No one to lean on, rely on or blame. The gift is yours – it is an amazing journey – and you alone are responsible for the quality of it.**"**
>
> *Dan Zadra/Bob Moaward*

You know that saying, "Go with your gut?" Well, it holds a special kind of truth for the health of your whole body. For years, you've been "listening to your gut" by using your intuition, so it may not surprise you that the system that controls your gut is also known as the "second brain," or the enteric nervous system (ENS).

The enteric nervous system can operate autonomously, like the coordination of reflexes. The ENS controls the various elements of your digestive system, like the conductor in a music hall. When all parts of the system work well together, the result is a beautiful symphony that leaves you feeling great; when elements of your digestive system are out of tune, this will affect your entire body. Through intestinal muscles, for example, the motor neurons in the ENS automatically control peristalsis, the involuntary constriction and relaxation of the muscles of the intestine, creating wavelike movement that pushes the contents of the canal forward, and churning of contents in the stomach. Not chewing one's food properly, not drinking enough water, lack of balance in the autonomic nervous system, and constantly feeling stressed can cause these muscles not to work properly, which also contributes to constipation or diarrhea. Additional neurons control secretion of enzymes.

Like the brain, the enteric nervous system also makes use of more than 30 neurotransmitters, such as acetylcholine, (cognition and memory), dopamine (motivation, cognition, and attention), and serotonin; a lack of dopamine causes mental and physical tiredness. More than 90% of the body's serotonin lies in the gut, as well as about 50% of the body's dopamine (Pasricha, 2011). And you thought this was all in your head! It's in your gut!

In addition to neurotransmitters, your gut also houses most of the immune system. Therefore, an unhealthy gut can cause problems throughout the rest of your body and your brain. When asked about their immune system, most people would not think of their gut. However, we have multiple species of bacteria that occupy the gut and comprise the natural flora, or good bacteria. These microbiota breakdown nutrients, prevent colonization of pathogenic bacteria, and can induce different types of immune cells and responses. This suggests that specific gut bacteria can affect disease development in organs other than the gut.

So how common are gut imbalances and issues? Consider these startling statistics. Proton pump inhibitors such as Prilosec and Prevacid (used to treat acid reflux disease) are the world's most popular drugs, accounting for $9.5 billion in sales in the US (Consumer Reports, 2013). 70 million Americans suffer from digestive issues such as indigestion, heartburn, irritable bowel syndrome, peptic and gastric ulcers, and Crohn's disease each day (Eisenstein, 2010). While the pharmaceutical industry offers prescriptions and over-the-counter remedies for gastrointestinal ailments, these 'solutions' are not without potentially serious side effects, and do not address the underlying causes of these digestive disorders.

Stress, poor dietary and lifestyle habits, bacterial infections, lack of beneficial intestinal flora, poor enzyme status, gut inflammation, and intestinal permeability (leaky gut), are some of the most common reasons for digestive distress. These problems are so common people often don't even realize they have them. For instance, I used to ask my clients if they were constipated and they would say "no". Turns out many of them were only having one bowel movement a week. This is constipation!

A bowel movement once a week is not healthy for the body as it allows waste to sit in your gut for days at a time during which toxins circulate through your bloodstream, causing inflammation and promoting the overgrowth of yeast and bacteria. Constipation also does not allow excess hormones to be eliminated from your body. Why? Excess estrogen, for example, is excreted in the bowel. When stool remains in the bowel for a longer period of time, the estrogen is reabsorbed. Women on a high fiber diet have lower levels of circulating estrogen. Less estrogen means less stimulation of breast tissue, which reduces the risk of breast cancer.

The Power of Healing Food Choices

Your digestive system is where the rest of your body gets its nutrients but it's also where toxins and germs often enter the body. What enters your gut affects everything from your brain, to your immune system, to your blood stream. This means that the key to managing many health problems starts in the gut.

Eating a whole foods diet and balancing blood sugar are habits that can produce profound health changes. By "whole foods" I don't mean you have to eat foods only from Whole Foods Market (though Whole Foods is a great place to shop), but that you eat food as close to nature as possible. This means avoiding foods that have been over-processed or genetically modified during food manufacturing.

Examples of overly manipulated foods are potato chips, snack bars, frozen dinners, jarred sauces, and condiments. Whole foods like fresh vegetables, fruits, nuts, and legumes retain the fiber and nutrients that are often removed in food processing. Eating a whole foods diet doesn't mean a boring diet, it means making healthier choices, like eating a homemade, baked chicken breast with savory herbs instead of frozen chicken nuggets processed with fats, fake flavorings, and chemical preservatives; or eating a real baked potato with green onions, instead of bagged potato chips with chemically-flavored onions. The more "retro" you eat (like your grandparents, before fast food), the healthier vanguard you will be.

Eating a whole foods diet is one of the best steps you can take to get your mojo back, but for some people, it's not enough. For complicated cases and for people suffering from chronic health complaints, I recommend initially embracing the anti-inflammatory diet, which I will discuss a little later.

Most Americans suffer from some degree of inflammation in their body, whether they realize it or not. Just because something doesn't hurt, doesn't mean it's not inflamed. Your gut or your brain can be inflamed, but they don't hurt because they have no pain fibers. Instead, symptoms such as brain fog, depression, food sensitivities, or hormonal imbalances show up to signal that something isn't right.

Although the primary goal of the anti-inflammatory diet is to tame inflammation and autoimmune attacks, a nice perk is that it's also a weight-loss diet for many. But weight loss shouldn't be your goal. A body struggling with significant imbalances will be reluctant to let go of excess weight until it can find balance, so focus on improving your health and decreasing inflammation in the body as your primary goals, and weight loss may naturally follow, Girlfriend! Wouldn't that be nice?

One of the most significant steps you can take to improve your health is to avoid one of the most common inflammatory substances in the modern American diet: gluten. If you are sensitive to gluten, it will eventually cause your immune system to attack and destroy your body, whether it's your gut, thyroid, joints, pancreas, or brain. Gluten is one of the biggest culprits I have seen in my office for causing autoimmune conditions, fibromyalgia, fatigue, neurological issues, and other chronic health problems. Gluten is in wheat, rye, oats, barley, spelt, and kamut.

The Benefits of Eliminating Gluten

Holly, 37 and a mother of two kids, came to see me because of migraines and low energy. "I feel like I am on the outside looking in at my own family because I don't have the health to be a real mom." You cannot raise children while contending with headaches and feeling tired. She said the straw that broke the camel's back was when her 12 year old said, "Mom, you are always tired, for my birthday do you think you will feel well enough to go on the outing the family has planned?"

Holly thought, of course, why not? Her daughter reminded her that the last two birthdays she had left the party early due to a migraine. Holly had totally forgotten this, and had thought she was doing a better job of hiding her fatigue. She didn't want her children to look back on their childhood and remember their mom being "sick" all the time. Holly went on a gluten-free diet, took magnesium, and a thyroid supplement that increases T3 and balanced out her insulin resistance. This reduced her migraines initially to twice a month, from once a week. After six months she had no migraines, her energy was boosted, and she was enjoying feeling part of her own family. "I feel like the mom again." As an added bonus, she lost 7 of the 10 lbs. that she had been struggling with.

Lucy, 52, sought relief from debilitating allergies. "It is so embarrassing, I am always blowing my nose at what seems like the most inconvenient times. Sunday in church my husband reached over and wiped a little dribble of snot from the bottom of my nose!" she said. She then added sarcastically, "I felt so feminine and grown up!"

Lucy had been taking several strong allergy medications for years. She began a gluten-free diet and eliminated refined foods, sodas, sugars and caffeine from her diet. She went on a natural antihistamine, quercetin, which is found in garlic and onions, repaired her gut with a protein shake high in glutamine, ginger, and turmeric, and started on specialized probiotics and digestive enzymes. Not only did a lifetime of severe allergies quickly disappear, but she also dropped 10 pounds and gained enough energy to start a Zumba class!

Laura, 28, was a Psychologist and had a very busy practice. She was planning a large wedding and came to see me because of fatigue, brain fog, constipation, and a lifelong rash on the back of her arms. "My life is so good, and I couldn't be happier. Yet, I am dragging around like I just lost my best friend. I don't seem to have energy after work to shop for the wedding, or make decisions about anything. I second guess what decisions I finally do make. All the wedding gowns are sleeveless and I don't want this rash to show. To boot, I am only having one bowel movement every four to five days!

I streamlined a gluten free lifestyle for Laura, added some adaptogens, adrenal support, magnesium, natural melatonin and GABA support. After 6 weeks the rash was *gone, she was reporting feeling more energetic, and was paying daily visits to the porcelain throne! She also reported being more decisive, having less brain fog, and was looking forward with optimism to her new season of life.*

Gluten can also cause weight gain due to the inflammation it causes. Dairy, eggs, yeast, corn, nuts, and soy are other common culprits causing inflammation. Normally, it is important for the body to use a short-term inflammation process to fight off infections and injuries. The presence of chronic, uncontrolled low-grade inflammation is an underlying factor in many disease states such as psoriasis, lupus, cardiovascular problems, and obesity. High blood sugar, high blood pressure, smoking, and chronic overeating can flip the inflammation switch on.

Chronic inflammation can cause you to become insulin resistant (insulin is the hormone that helps control blood sugar) and leptin resistant (leptin is a hormone that makes you feel satiated); both of these conditions lead to increased appetite and weight gain. When you eat inflammatory foods, an immune reaction is initiated; when you continue to eat them, you develop chronic inflammation in the body, which in turn can contribute to weight gain. I have a client who was already on a gluten-free diet, but when she quit eating dairy she immediately dropped 15 pounds. This was a clear sign that her immune system had been reacting negatively to dairy products for years.

Your health and comfort are not a guessing game; when you're having serious health issues you need to be tested to determine if you're reactive to gluten. The testing should include the different components of gluten that people react to, as most standard labs only test for one, alpha gliadin. **A test that only screens for alpha gliadin will misdiagnose many people.** The only lab I know of right now that runs the test for all the components of gluten is Cyrex Labs (visit www.ThyroSisters.com for more info on them). I have yet to have a client with an autoimmune disorder who is not sensitive to gluten, and often they are sensitive to other foods as well. This is why the autoimmune diet is so helpful. The restrictive nature of the diet helps build dietary focus and control, both are important skills when you have a chronic immune condition.

Introducing the Anti-Inflammatory Diet

Approach this new way of eating and staying healthy with an attitude of abundance, not deprivation or fear, and keep in mind the importance of not eating any of the foods on the "Foods to Avoid" list. Even just a small snack or a little bite can trigger inflammation and sabotage all your hard work. The initial cravings will pass quickly, especially as you start to feel and function so much better.

Foods to Eat

- **Most organic vegetables.** The exceptions are white potatoes because they are too starchy and can spike blood sugar. Also avoid corn (which is technically a grain) and nightshades (tomatoes, eggplant, peppers), which provoke inflammation in some people.
- **Fermented and cultured foods.** The Specific Carbohydrate Diet (SCD) and Gut and Psychology Syndrome (GAPS) diets in particular promote the gut-healing properties of fermented foods, which contain "good" bacteria for your gut. Examples include kimchi, kombucha tea, pickled ginger, sauerkraut, and unsweetened coconut yogurt. Make your own or buy one of the few brands that are genuinely fermented (not made with vinegar) and free of sugars or additives.
- **Meats.** Fish should be coldwater fish, and wild, with a low mercury content. If possible, buy pastured and organic meats from a local reputable farm or online. Second best is buying organic from the store. Avoid factory-farmed meats that contain antibiotics and hormones.
- **Low glycemic organic fruits.** Choose fruits that are mildly sweet, such as berries or plums, and eat in moderation. As a rule of thumb, choose fruits with a pit in them, they are usually lower in sugar, good choices are apricots and plums vs. grapes or bananas.
- **Coconut.** Coconut milk, coconut butter, coconut cream, coconut oil, unsweetened coconut flakes, and homemade unsweetened coconut yogurt are all options. Coconut milk in cans and cartons contain thickening agents that may be problematic for some people. You may be able to find filler-

free coconut milk or cream in the frozen section of an Asian grocery store. Note: Although coconut is popular today, some people react to it, so pay attention to your symptoms and avoid if necessary.

- **Herbs and spices.** Basil, black pepper, cilantro, coriander, cumin, garlic, ginger, lemongrass, mint, oregano, parsley, rosemary, sage, sea salt, thyme.
- **Other:** apple cider vinegar, herbal teas, olive oil, and olives.

Foods to Avoid

- Very **sweet fruits**, such as pineapple, banana, or dried fruits.
- **All grains**, including corn, which is found in many processed foods.
- **Spices and Condiments:** It is common for gluten to hide in commercial salad dressings, Ketchup, curry powder, horseradish sauces, soy sauce (except Tamari), imitation seafood, instant hot drinks (coffee, hot chocolate), veined cheeses, bouillon cubes, MSG (Monosodium Glutamate, a flavor enhancer), and rice syrup. Check that these items are labeled "Gluten Free."
- All **sugars and sweeteners**, including the natural and so-called low-glycemic ones.
- **All dairy**, including cow, sheep, and goat dairy. Instead substitute rice, or coconut milk.
- **Eggs** and all products containing eggs, such as mayonnaise. This includes duck, goose, and quail eggs. Even free-range eggs can be problematic. If the chickens eat GMO grains, so do you, and you may react negatively.
- **All soy.** Watch for soy hidden in other ingredients.
- **Nightshades.** These are pro-inflammatory for many people and include potatoes, sweet and hot peppers, tomatoes, eggplants, and spices derived from peppers.
- Some people may want to avoid **mushrooms** and other fungi if they have Candida overgrowth.
- **Alcohol.** Most alcohol is made from grains or other inflammatory foods, like grapes. Alcohol also contains a lot of complex sugars, which are also inflammatory.

- **Beans and legumes.** Legumes contain phytic acid. Phytic acid binds to nutrients in food, preventing you from absorbing them. Beans and legumes also contain a type of carbohydrate called galaco-oligosaccharides that cause unpleasant digestive problems for some people, such as irritable bowel syndrome.
- **Processed foods.** These often have hidden inflammatory foods, like gluten, corn, and soy.

COMMON QUESTIONS ABOUT THE ANTI-INFLAMMATORY DIET

1. **Why no grains, legumes, or sweeteners?**
   Grains, legumes, and all sweeteners (except honey) contain disaccharides or polysaccharides, complex sugars that feed the harmful bacteria contributing to leaky gut and inflammation. Grains also trigger a reaction in many people who are gluten-intolerant. Other foods that commonly cause inflammation include dairy, chocolate, sesame, and instant coffee.

2. **When can I start re-introducing foods?**
   Some people come to love this diet and stick to it as a way of life, because it has given them their health back. Others may find they can reintroduce some, or many, of the foods that are initially restricted. You have the freedom to choose what is best for you, you're a brilliant, intuitive ThyroSister! From what you are learning in this book and experiencing in making lifestyle changes, you have re-connected your mind-body, and can trust your intuitive judgment.

   One goal of the diet is to find out which foods cause inflammation, and this can vary from person to person. To figure this out, reintroduce foods in a systematic manner. Reintroduce the restricted foods one at a time every 72 hours, and closely monitor for reactions.

Reactions can include joint pain, skin rashes or eruptions, fatigue, brain fog, mood swings, gut pain or problems, chest congestion, runny nose, and others. It totally depends on the person, so pay attention and keep a journal; you may discover something in terms of food sensitivities that can change your life.

3. **Are there ways to supplement the autoimmune diet?**
    This diet is some powerful mojo on its own. However, for tough cases I also suggest using several nutritional compounds developed by Dr. Kharrazian and other nutritional pioneers, to tame inflammation and help restore gut health. These include therapeutic doses of highly absorbable resveratrol and curcumin, probiotics, digestive enzymes, HCl (to boost stomach acid) and ox bile extract to support the gallbladder (if necessary). Bile acids are produced from cholesterol in your liver and then flow into your gallbladder where they are stored and concentrated. As your body senses the movement of fat into the small intestines the gallbladder releases the bile to emulsify the fat, making it easier to absorb.

    There are also great gut repair nutrients to include L-glutamine, deglycyrrhizinated licorice extract, aloe vera, marshmallow extract, slippery elm extract, gamma oryzanol, MSM, and Spanish moss. These are herbs that can be found separately in health food stores, or in one combined formula from your health care professional. Working with a knowledgeable health care practitioner will help guide you through the nuances of repairing the gut.

    To further improve your understanding of how to heal your gut and why it's so important to do so, here's more about the most common gut disorders, and ways to treat them effectively.

Common Gut Disorders

- ## *Leaky Gut*

  The autoimmune diet helps to repair leaky gut, a disorder previously discussed. It actually is as awful as it sounds. When you eat a poor diet (including too much sugar) and have chronic stress or blood sugar imbalances, you are at high risk of developing leaky gut. This means the wall of your small intestine, which absorbs nutrients from food, becomes inflamed, damaged, and overly porous. Undigested foods, bacteria, yeast, and other 'nasties' spill through the gut wall into the bloodstream. The immune system sees this as an invasion and deploys its 'soldiers' to attack and destroy the invaders.

  Unfortunately, when your gut is damaged this can happen every time you eat, which keeps your immune system on constant red alert. Eventually the immune system starts attacking your body tissue, keeping your gut and your body in a constant state of inflammation. Researchers have also discovered that leaky gut can lead to inflammation in the brain; causing schizophrenia, memory loss, brain lesions, and an increased risk of dementia and Parkinson's (Kharrazian). In fact, it's now accepted that gut inflammation is a common cause of depression and other mental and mood disorders (Bested AC, 2013). **Repairing a leaky gut is vital to restoring your health and is the primary aim of the autoimmune diet.**

- ## *Bacterial Infections in the Gut*

  Sometimes the gut becomes so weakened that it is besieged by an overgrowth of infectious bacteria. One of the most common infections is a Helicobacter pylori overgrowth. H.pylori is a spiral shaped bacterium commonly found in the stomach. The way the bacteria moves allows them to penetrate the stomach's protective lining, where they produce substances that weaken the lining and make the stomach more susceptible to damage from gastric acids. The bacteria can attach to cells of the stomach, causing inflammation and creating excess stomach acid. It is not really known how H.pylori infection is spread, but scientists believe it may be contracted through contaminated food and water.

These bacteria can cause low stomach acid, poor digestion, and ulcers. Some scientists believe that H. pylori is the most commonly transmitted disease in the world. Ingredients to combat this infection include Golden Seal, Barberry extract, Oregon grape root, Chinese goldthread, and Yerba mansa. Cranberry, 400 mg twice a day, has been shown in preliminary research to possibly reduce Helicobacter pylori.

Some people have parasites, such as worms or amoebas, and don't know it. You don't have to live in a third-world country to get parasites. Parasite eggs are often microscopic and can be virtually anywhere. This includes lakes and rivers, restrooms, on animals (even house pets), undercooked meats, and unwashed fruits and vegetables. These critters like to gobble up B-vitamins, which depletes your energy. An overgrowth of harmful bacteria in the gut can also decrease the amount of calories you're able to absorb from your food. In these cases it may be necessary to purge the gut with some powerful herbs and nutrients.

Garlic has been known to have activity against roundworm (Ascaris). Goldenseal (Hydrastis Canadensis) has been used for infections of the mucous membranes in the body, such as the respiratory tract. Black walnut is a folk herbal remedy used for ringworm and athlete's foot. Pumpkin seeds have been used as a remedy for tapeworms and roundworms. Whew! Fun stuff crawling around in our guts, huh? If there still seem to be symptoms of an infection after the cleanse, I order a stool panel that screens for many different harmful bacteria, yeast, and parasites. It's called GI Effects and is available from Genova/ Metametrix.

- *Hydrochloric Acid Deficiency*

Many people who are vegetarians, or not used to eating meat, are deficient in hydrochloric acid (HCI), a stomach acid needed to digest proteins. If you feel sick or heavy after eating meat, this is likely due to a poor ability to digest meat. Many people today become deficient in hydrochloric acid, especially as they age. This is especially true for those who eat heavily cooked foods, foods that are difficult to digest such as fried foods, foods containing artificial preservatives and additives, soft drinks, and blackened foods (the blackened areas of the food contain cancer-causing agents). Antibiotics, painkillers, and excessive alcohol are other factors that can deplete stomach acid. Those with poor stomach acid typically have low Vitamin C levels as well.

Thirty percent of people aged 60 and over suffer from low acid secretion, and forty percent of postmenopausal women have no basal gastric acid secretions at all. (English, 2013). If this is the case for you, taking a hydrochloric acid supplement (HCL) can radically improve the health and chemistry of your digestive tract. The parietal cells of the stomach produce HCL, mostly in response to ingested protein or fat. Stress can also stimulate acid output. Decreased HCL production causes gas, bloating, and discomfort after rich meals. Furthermore, you may have difficulty absorbing minerals like iron and calcium, leading to conditions to include iron deficiency anemia and osteoporosis. Diabetics tend to have lower secretion of HCL, as do people with eczema, psoriasis, and periodontal disease.

A hydrochloric acid supplement is available as betaine hydrochloride. When a 64mg capsule is taken before, during, or after a meal, it should help break down peptides and amino acids and fats into triglycerides. Betaine can be used alone or with other digestive agents, such as pepsin. Be cautious, however, if you know you have an ulcer, gastritis or excessive stomach acid because HCL will have a tendency to irritate the condition.

Drinking the juice of half a lemon in water, or a teaspoon of apple cider vinegar in warm water may correct low stomach acid as well. Also rosemary, ginger, cumin, and orange peel, made into a tea, have been shown to be helpful. Taking niacin, B3 and B6 can also help to stimulate HCL production. HCL can help kill off bad bacteria and other pathogens, protect your gut from ingested bacteria, improve nutrient absorption, trigger the release of necessary digestive chemicals, and improve bowel function.

Hydrochloric acid is one of your body's first-line defenses against disease-causing microbes. Weak stomach acid allows infecting organisms (normally killed by the acid), to get past the stomach and set up infections in other areas.

How Low Stomach Acid Causes Heartburn

If you go to your healthcare provider and say, "I have acid reflux, I keep burping, and I'm bloated after eating," you'll most likely get a prescription for a proton pump inhibitor (PPI). PPI's work by suppressing the molecules responsible for the release of stomach acid, you may be familiar with names such as Nexium, Prilosec, and Protonix. **But the reason you have acid reflux is not because you have too much acid in your stomach; it is because you don't have enough, and what is available is in the wrong place.** I know! This is a real jaw dropping statement! Opposite to what you have heard which is that you have too much acid in the gut and that is causing reflux.

Taking a PPI will drive your stomach acid levels even lower. This provides an initial period of symptom relief, but makes the overall problem even worse. So what is causing the burning sensation? The burning in your esophagus and throat is due to the fermenting and putrefying food in your stomach washing back up into your esophagus. When stomach acid is low, it cannot properly digest the food. Various messenger chemicals in the gut depend on sufficient stomach acidity to trigger the passage of food from the stomach into the small intestine. If the acidity is too low, then these chemicals are not activated and the food sits in the stomach, eventually moving back up into the esophagus.

If you've struggled with Gerd, bloating, or acid reflex you've probably been given a long list of foods to avoid, like greasy foods, spicy foods, and chocolate. You might be surprised to learn that avoiding these foods improves symptoms in some people but not a lot! The easiest way to find out if these foods negatively impact you is to eliminate them from your diet for 6 weeks, then reintroduce one at a time.

A better approach is this: eat foods high in B vitamins and calcium, like raw almonds and dark leafy vegetables, such as spinach and kale. Eat less red meat and more coldwater fish or beans for protein. Avoid refined foods, especially white breads and sugary packaged foods. Eliminate trans fatty acids found in cookies, crackers, French fries, and doughnuts. Carbonated drinks, coffee and alcohol all irritate the stomach lining.

Taking Omega-3 fatty acids such as fish oil, (1 tablespoon 2 or 3 times a day) may help decrease inflammation, but don't take any if you are on blood thinning meds. (Choose omega-3 fatty acids products where the majority of Vitamin A has been removed to avoid a toxic overload.) Probiotic supplements containing Lactobacillus acidophilus, a friendly bacteria, may help maintain balance in your digestive tract.

DGL-licorice (Glycyrrhiza Glabra) is an herb that may protect against damage from NSAIDS (non-steroidal anti-inflammatory drugs) like ibuprofen, aspirin, and Naproxen. A peppermint (Mentha Piperita) standardized 1 tablet with meals may relieve symptoms of a peptic ulcer. Losing weight, if you need to, is an effective way of controlling acid reflex as well. Wearing tight clothes, exercising after eating, or lying down after a meal, all put pressure on the lower esophageal sphincter (LES).

Being faithful to this new lifestyle will really pay off if you've been suffering from heartburn or bloating. You will enjoy freedom from pain, bad breath, fatigue, hoarseness and throat clearing. Left unchecked, too much acid in the wrong place can cause precancerous changes called Barrett's esophagus, hip fractures, (due to mal-absorption of calcium from being on chronic PPI's), as well as respiratory diseases and tooth decay (Moe GL, 2006).

HELPFUL HINT!

Make sure you are getting an adequate daily intake of salt, from natural sea salt to include Mediterranean Sea salt, or Himalayan salt. The chloride fraction contained in high-quality salt is essential for your body to make hydrochloric acid.

Don't Neglect These Important Organs

Two important digestive organs we sometimes forget about are the liver and gallbladder. The liver detoxifies the blood, and the gallbladder secretes bile to help digest fats. **For perimenopausal and menopausal women the liver is especially important, because it helps detoxify the body of excess and unneeded hormones.** When the liver becomes sluggish, toxic metabolites of estrogen can get too high, causing symptoms such as fatigue, weight gain, and brain fog, and also raising the risk of cancers, due to estrogen dominance. Therefore, I like to keep female patients with hormonal imbalances on liver and gallbladder support that includes dandelion root, milk thistle seed extract, trimethylglycine, N-acetyl L-cysteine, Gotu kola, Cordyceps, beet, L-glutamine, phospholipids, taurine, ginger, glycine, DL-methionine, alpha lipoic acid, choline, betaine HCl, panax ginseng, MSM, and enzymes.

Many of my clients decide to use a protein shake that includes many nutritional compounds to gently cleanse and detox the liver and gut on a daily basis. Although there are many protein shake formulas out there, my favorites are formulated with high amounts of L- Glutamine, N-Acetyl-L-Cysteine, Alpha Lipoic Acid and turmeric. These substances help to decrease inflammation, and repair the tight junctions that have broken open in the digestive tract. One version is made with rice protein, and another with pea protein, if you find you cannot tolerate grains. They are all surprisingly tasty and work well to maintain the health of these important organs. You can add these healing protein powders into delicious smoothies for a meal replacement, or a pick-me-up, see www.ThyroSisters.com for great recipe ideas.

Enzymes Support Better Digestion

Efficient digestion will help to enhance your immune system's response. With good digestion the body can destroy harmful organisms naturally present in food, before they gain entry to the body. This saves the body from many potential infections. Good digestion also prevents the entry of poorly digested food particles into the blood. Achieving efficient digestion results in a healthier gut, lower cholesterol, improved mineral absorption, better blood sugar levels, lower triglycerides, and even the prevention of tooth decay.

In contrast, poor digestion leads the body to become more toxic and inflamed, and can lead to fatigue, aching joints, skin disorders, hypersensitivity reactions, and allergies. Poorly digested food particles will over activate the immune system and cause chronic inflammation.

Exciting new research suggests that taking plant-based enzymes with meals can slow the aging process, enhance the immune response, reduce inflammation, and improve digestion – thereby extending the life of your own enzyme system (Donaldson, 2011). But you need to be aware of 'junk enzymes'. The digestive enzymes used in commercial digestive products vary widely in quality. When it comes to enzymes look for good quality ones. Even if they are more expensive, they're worth it. How do you know if an enzyme is quality? First the most important measurement is the activity and potency, not the weight or milligrams. There's a national standard for the evaluation of enzymes and it comes from the Food Chemical Codex, (FCC).

Enzymes are catalysts that enable molecules to be changed from one form to another. For example, digestive enzymes enable food to be broken down to produce energy. Plant-based digestive enzymes have the nutrients necessary for our bodies to maximize digestion of the fruits and veggies we eat. Vitamins do not deliver energy by themselves, they require enzymes for energy. Enzymes unlock the energy in food and make it possible for the human body to function properly. Proteins, sugars, starches, and fats require specific types of enzymes to be broken down properly, so when taking supplements it's best to get a formula that will work on everything. Amylase enzyme works on starches, lactase on milk sugars, protease on proteins, and lipase on fats. A good formula will contain all of these enzymes.

Hormone Health Depends on Nutritional Health

If your hormones are out of whack, it's imperative to support your body with a high quality diet. Hormonal imbalances are extremely stressful on the body and raise the risk for many chronic health conditions. The great news is that some women have been able to completely resolve symptoms of hormonal imbalance by following the anti-inflammatory diet and repairing their leaky gut. Others still may need bio-identical hormone therapy, but will get better results, and with lower doses, by eating well too. Food is either your medicine or your poison. Eat healthy for a high quality, mojo-filled life. I've helped many people transition to better health through dietary recommendations, education, and support. If you are not perfect on this diet, it's okay! Be kind to yourself. It's not how many times you fall, it's how many times you get back up that counts!

Ask your health professional to run a GI Effects Stool Profile from Genova/Metametrex Clinical Laboratory. This is the latest advancement in stool analysis for truly comprehensive results.

Secrets Whispered to a ThyroSister

Other reasons your gut may be functioning poorly

In evaluating how well or how poorly your gut functions, it is also important to be tested for parasites, as they can play a role in autoimmune diseases. Many people suffer from parasites and don't know it. A lot of people who suffer from Hashimoto's or fibromyalgia also suffer from IBS (irritable bowel syndrome) and experience problems with constipation, diarrhea, or both.

- Join our community of ThyroSisters at www.ThyroSisters.com where you will find tips on gut repair, gluten free recipes, and cutting edge information on supplements and improving gut health.

- AVOID taking NSAIDs. Non-steroidal anti-inflammatory drugs such as Advil, Motrin, and Aleve make leaky gut worse. Keep in mind that you will not need to take anti-inflammatory medication once you restore your health.

- If you suffer from heartburn or acid reflux, consider taking an HCl supplement and high quality digestive enzymes. You need to take HCl and enzymes separately. I recommend taking enzymes 10 - 20 minutes before the meal and HCl during the meal. (Do not take digestive enzymes or HCl if you have an ulcer.)

- If you want more specific information about what foods you need to avoid, you can test for reactivity with gluten-associated sensitivity panels and cross reactive foods (found at www.ThyroSisters.com) which test for reactivity to the following foods: *spelt, barley, rye, polish wheat, milk proteins, milk chocolate, oats, yeast, instant coffee, oats, sesame, buckwheat, sorghum, millet, hemp, amaranth, quinoa, tapioca, teff, soy, egg, corn, rice, potato.* If you test positive to any of these foods, then you know you need to avoid them. How long you will need to do so depends on other health factors, such as whether you are managing autoimmune or other chronic conditions.

CHAPTER 7
BUILDING TO SCALE:
Resolving Weight Problems

> **"** It's bizarre that the produce manager is more important to my children's health than the pediatrician. **"**
>
> *Meryl Streep*

Many women beat themselves up for being overweight, when the real reason for putting on pounds is not over-eating but poor thyroid function, food intolerances, autoimmune issues, inflammation, hormonal imbalance, or a brain chemistry imbalance. While crash dieting and exercise can help with weight loss, addressing the root causes that contribute to excess weight will bring lasting, healthy results.

The difference between most dieting approaches and a functional protocol approach is that the latter will naturally restore your health, including the return to a well-functioning metabolism. In many cases, excess weight is a symptom of an underlying health problem. You need to identify and address this issue before starting a weight loss program that will be effective and have lasting results.

Julie came to see me because of exhaustion, and had been diagnosed with fibromyalgia. She couldn't sleep, even though she felt tired all the time. The mother of two children in grade school, she worked part-time and was very involved in her community and church activities: all good things that make up an enriching life, but

Julie felt overwhelmed. Stress was a constant companion. "My husband tells me to eat less and exercise more." To add to her exasperation, Julie had been on several diets in an attempt to lose weight, with no success. "I get up early and exercise for 90-minutes, five days a week!" she exclaimed, throwing her hands in the air. She was also limiting her food intake to mostly vegetables, a little fruit, and a small amount of protein. "I had my thyroid checked and it came back normal. And I haven't lost a single ounce! My workout partner has lost 10 pounds!"

I worked with Julie on a three-month program, and she lost 28 pounds. In evaluating her situation we took a step-by-step approach to identify the underlying causes of her fatigue and inability to lose weight, in spite of doing 'everything right.'

There are health issues that contribute to weight gain; here are the most common culprits that can put on unwanted pounds.

- Poorly functioning thyroid
- Undiagnosed intolerances to food
- Elevated insulin levels (from too many sugars and carbohydrates in the diet)
- Cells deprived of oxygen
- High or low cortisol levels
- Hormone imbalances
- Not enough stomach acid
- Neurotransmitters out of balance
- Not getting enough quality sleep

Real Help for Stubborn Weight Loss

• *Thyroid Issues*

Poor thyroid function is a common cause of weight gain, because the thyroid regulates metabolism. Like Julie, you may have had your thyroid checked, and were told you are "normal." Your friends and family may think you're using your thyroid as an excuse for not reaching your weight loss goals. Perhaps you've heard the advice, "exercise more, and eat less." Well, that works if your whole body biochemistry is functioning normally. Let's face this head on, Girlfriend, we all know how to diet; what you are learning in this new season in your life is how to eat, embrace abundance, and maintain a healthy weight.

I don't like diets! They perpetuate self-loathing. Think about it: all the negative self-talk, beating yourself up, judging your self-worth by the scale, and comparing yourself to others that have a different biochemistry. Frustrated and discouraged, it's easy to go back to old habits, thinking, "I am such a loser, have no self-control, and if I would just exercise more and eat less like Veronica Voom Voom, I would achieve my goals and finally be happy!"

Well, let's take a fresh look at this weight loss thing. And no, you don't have to live on kale and wheatgrass juice to have success. When the thyroid gland starts to fail, metabolism slows and weight gain increases. I've heard many stories from women who followed a strict diet and exercised daily, yet packed on pounds because of an undiagnosed thyroid condition. This is frustrating and can be a serious blow to self-esteem and efforts to be healthy.

There is an interesting, yet complex relationship between low thyroid, body weight, and metabolism. Hormones produced in the thyroid regulate your metabolism, so if your thyroid underperforms, your body metabolism will not burn fast enough. Often slow metabolism makes it nearly impossible to lose weight, and often causes weight gain. We can measure how well your metabolism is functioning by measuring the amount of oxygen used by the body over a specific amount of time. If the measurement is made at rest, it's called basal metabolic rate (BMR). Patients whose thyroid glands are producing low output are associated with low BMR. The BMR is subject to many other influences, so further tests may be necessary to pinpoint the underlying issue.

Conventional wisdom tells us that in order to maintain body weight, we need to burn as many calories as we eat each day, this is called achieving energy balance. So you would think that if you ate fewer calories, and burned more fuel, you would lose weight. Au contraire, Mon Ami Girlfriend, there are other hormones such as progesterone, proteins, and chemicals to include cortisol and insulin that influence energy expenditure. These substances interact with the brain centers that regulate energy, and influence tissues in the body.

In controlling energy expenditure and energy intake, you need to be mindful that there are many variables working in concert to keep your body balanced. But don't worry. We are going to look at all the tools you can use to achieve your ideal weight.

Remember Julie? It turns out she had only been tested for one out of six possible variables of thyroid performance: TSH, thyroid stimulating hormone. I ordered a more in-depth test that revealed her thyroid was indeed at the root of her health issues. But perhaps I hear you saying, *"I've been on thyroid medication, and I still can't lose weight!"* I frequently hear this complaint. The reason is that you have been tested and treated for only one variable of thyroid performance. Instead, you need to evaluate not just your TSH level, but also a number of other factors: *Is your thyroid effectively converting T4 to T3? Is the pituitary gland correctly sending signals to the thyroid? Are adequate levels of neurotransmitters being made in the gut to signal the hypothalamus, to then signal the pituitary gland, to make TSH?* A thorough evaluation is needed to answer these questions and to determine the best approach to getting your thyroid back on track.

• *Food Intolerances*

If more in-depth thyroid tests come back normal, don't give up! There's something else at the root of those stubborn muffin-tops, and we're going to find out what it is! When it comes to weight gain, sensitivities to gluten, casein (a protein in milk), eggs, and other food allergies must be ruled out. If you are sensitive to certain foods, this will be very gratifying for you, because you will see such dramatic, lasting improvement, without drugs.

An allergy, or chronic sensitivity, is an over-reaction of the immune system, the body's natural defense system. Women may suffer transient, seemingly disconnected symptoms that can be difficult to recognize. In a protective effort, your body goes on red alert. Thinking it's under attack, it starts releasing antibodies and triggering inflammation. Inflammation is a process by which the body's white blood cells and chemicals protect us from infection with foreign substances, such as bacteria and viruses.

Like a row of dominoes, the allergic response engages the body's inflammatory cascade, which causes serious health effects, like mood disorders, skin rashes, and respiratory ailments. Whether the allergic response is an "allergy" or "sensitivity" is merely a matter of degree; either way, your body will become inflamed. If your body is alerting you to a problem through symptoms, you probably have some kind of sensitivity, even if the allergy tests keep coming back normal. Take measures to alleviate your body's allergic reaction or sensitivities. If you don't, your body will up the ante until you have full blown, chronic inflammation.

To start lightening the toxic load on your body, the most effective place to make positive changes is in your diet. A gluten-free diet, for example, often leads to a quick drop in weight, due in part to the reduction in carbohydrate intake by avoiding breads, pastas, and cereals. On the other hand, chronic overeating can cause hyperglycemia; high blood sugar. This can flip the inflammation switch on, causing insulin resistance. Insulin is crucial for balancing blood sugar and also regulates a hormone called leptin that is involved with satiety. Leptin imbalances can cause increased appetite and weight gain.

Even though wheat, rye, oats and barley look, taste, and smell the same as back in the day, the seeds that go into the ground these days are chemically treated and manufactured. Your body sees those chemicals as invaders and decides to inflame against them. So when genetically modified foods such as gluten, dairy, yeast, corn, nuts or soy cause an immune reaction in the body, inflammation occurs in an effort to protect you, and as a result often causes weight gain.

A patient who was already on a gluten-free diet quit eating dairy at my suggestion. She quickly dropped 15 pounds, a strong sign that her body's immune system was reacting to the dairy in her diet. It's a good idea to test for food sensitivities so you're clear about what foods trigger inflammation in your body. Find out through testing if you are intolerant to gluten or other foods, so you can avoid eating these foods. In addition, addressing these issues will also help improve energy so you feel more motivated to exercise.

• *Insulin Resistance*

In addition to an underperforming thyroid and inflammation, believe it or not, insulin resistance also makes shedding weight more difficult. Insulin is a hormone that opens the doors of the cell so that glucose (sugar) can leave the blood stream and enter into the cells.

Once in the cell, it is used to produce much-needed energy. Insulin resistance occurs when the cells of the body no longer respond well to insulin and don't allow sugars to pass through the cell membrane. When this happens, excess glucose stays in your bloodstream and causes elevated blood sugar levels. The body then turns these sugars into fat for storage. Excess calories from starch and sugar are the leading trigger for developing insulin resistance.

Muffin tops aren't the only problem with insulin resistance, however, and prolonged resistance leads to much bigger problems. Because the body does not like blood sugar levels to be elevated, the pancreas responds by churning out more and more insulin into the bloodstream, which basically forces the cell doors to open, so that more sugar can leave the blood stream and enter into the cells to help produce energy. In the early stages of insulin resistance, the insulin levels will be elevated, but the blood sugar levels will remain in the normal range. Over the course of decades, however, your body will build up a resistance to insulin. In the same way an alcoholic has to drink increasing amounts of alcohol to get drunk, your cells will require increasing amounts of insulin to be persuaded to take in even normal or low amounts of sugar.

Eventually, elevated insulin levels will no longer be able to effectively lower the blood sugar levels and your fasting blood sugar will start to rise. At this stage, full-blown diabetes is on the horizon. The simplest way to make the diagnosis of insulin resistance is by checking a fasting insulin level, with a blood test. A level greater than 10 indicates the early stages of insulin resistance, or what we call pre-diabetes. Elevated insulin levels can precede the development of full blown diabetes by 10 to 20 years.

A fasting blood sugar level above 99 is considered hyperglycemia, or high blood sugar.

These are the symptoms you might experience if you have insulin resistance:

- Fatigue after meals
- General fatigue
- Constant hunger
- Craving for sweets that isn't relieved by eating them
- Waist girth equal to or larger than hip girth
- Frequent urination
- Increased appetite and thirst
- Difficulty losing weight
- Migrating aches and pains

• *Reactive Hypoglycemia*

When your blood glucose falls precipitously, it's an instinct to reach for a sugary snack. Most likely, that snack will be calorie-dense, not nutrient-dense. Hypoglycemia occurs when your blood sugar repeatedly drops too low in response to eating sugary (high-carbohydrate) foods, or going too long without eating. If you thought starving yourself was a good way to diet, think again! Repeated episodes of hypoglycemia can lead to adrenal fatigue, which can also cause low blood sugar, creating a vicious downward spiral.

These are the most common symptoms of hypoglycemia.

- Craving sweets
- Irritability if you miss a meal
- Dependency on coffee for energy
- Becoming lightheaded if you miss a meal
- Eating to relieve fatigue
- Feeling shaky, jittery, or tremulous
- Feeling agitated or nervous
- Easily upset
- Poor memory, forgetfulness
- Blurred vision

Eating tips for blood-sugar imbalances

If your blood sugar is low and you experience symptoms of low blood sugar (to include shakiness, anxiety, sweating) missing meals is a habit you need to break. Start your day with healthy protein and fat, such as a veggie omelet with avocado and salsa, or almond butter on gluten free toast, or a protein smoothie made with almond milk. Eat a healthy snack every two to three hours. A person with hypoglycemia should never fast since it will make the problem even worse.

With hyperglycemia people feel sleepy or crave sugar after eating, especially after eating too many carbohydrates. If you feel sleepy after a low or no carbohydrate meal, you will need additional support with nutrients that help reverse insulin resistance.

If your blood sugar level is below 85, it is important that you eat every two to three hours to help keep blood sugar stable. You don't have to eat a whole meal, just a few bites of a healthy snack, vegetables, nuts, or seeds between meals, and a light snack before bed. If you do not have sugar-handling issues, it is best to eat three meals a day and not snack

• *Anemia*

When a client comes to me with symptoms of hypothyroidism, wanting to lose weight, and their blood tests don't show the usual antibodies that suggest an autoimmune condition, the next most likely suspect is anemia.

Anemia means that you either have a low number of red blood cells or that your red blood cells don't contain enough hemoglobin, an iron-rich protein that helps blood cells carry oxygen throughout the body.

Oxygen is life. It fuels your muscles, brain, metabolism, and organs. When you are low on red blood cells or hemoglobin, your body isn't getting enough oxygen. Think about how tired you'd feel if you could only fill your lungs up halfway with each breath. That's what's happening to your muscles, brain, and metabolism when you have anemia. As a result, you'll often feel weak, cold, shaky, and mentally dull. Work outs, if any, are not as robust as they used to be. Do these symptoms sound familiar? These are many of the symptoms of hypothyroidism!

The common "cure" for anemia is iron supplementation, but that isn't always the right solution. Some forms of anemia don't respond to iron supplementation, and they can actually make the condition worse by breaking down red blood cells, too much iron in the body can be constipating and toxic.

When I encounter a client who does not have an autoimmune condition, but despite a low calorie diet has not had much weight loss, I immediately test for anemia, blood sugar, gut/liver function, and fatty acid metabolism. Usually the culprit is in one of these categories.

• *Imbalanced Cortisol*

Remember all the stress you might have put on yourself to lose weight? Well, ThyroSister, I've got some bad news. Stressing out about your weight actually makes it harder to shed any pounds at all. High levels of cortisol associated with stress cause water retention, most likely because of an increase in aldosterone production. Aldosterone is an adrenal hormone that regulates how the body manages water. This also negatively impacts thyroid function, which can slow your metabolism. High cortisol is typically also linked with insulin resistance, which promotes fat storage and inhibits fat burning.

Low cortisol levels, on the other hand, lead to frequent drops in blood sugar, causing you to reach for sugary snacks to bring blood sugar back up. If this happens too often, your body may go into starvation mode, holding onto more of everything that you put in.

• *High or Low Testosterone*

Testosterone imbalances are another common cause of weight gain. Low testosterone in women can lead to poor mood, low energy, depression and loss of muscle mass -- all of which make it tough to stick to a healthy eating and activity plan. However, elevated testosterone levels can also cause problems, like hair loss and growth of facial hair. If testosterone levels are either too low or too high, it will be extremely difficult to feel at your best. Our constant enemy, stress, can lower testosterone, lower estrogen, and increase insulin.

For women, the most common imbalance is too much testosterone and too much cortisol, often a result of high-carbohydrate diets and lack of exercise. Not only does excess testosterone cause hair loss and growth of facial hair, but it also promotes stubborn belly fat (ever notice how men tend to get a beer belly instead of chunky arms and thighs like we ladies do?) As long as cortisol and testosterone levels are high, it will be extremely difficult to lose excess fat.

• *Excess Estrogen*

To lose fat you need both a caloric deficit and hormonal balance. Don't think of hormones working in isolation; they affect every system in our bodies. For example, an estrogen/progesterone imbalance has a tendency to make women store belly fat. Too much estrogen (estrogen dominance), causes excess fat storage, and often occurs in tandem with problems regulating blood sugar and insulin, or adrenal gland problems.

The cause is usually low progesterone, or an imbalance in the ratio of estrogen/progesterone that causes the body to lean towards fat storage. How does this happen? Two ways: we either produce too much estrogen on our own; or we acquire it from the environment or diet. Accumulating estrogen is easy to do, you are exposed to estrogen-like compounds in foods that contain toxic pesticides, herbicides, and growth hormones. These toxins cause weight gain, which fuels more production of estrogen in your fat cells.

Hormone replacement therapy (HRT) or birth control pills can increase estrogen as well. Estrogen has also been found in our drinking water and fertilizers that make the golf courses green and the grapes at the winery bigger. Non-organic dairy and meats, plastics, and non-GMO vegetables contain particles of estrogen, too.

So how do you know if you have too much estrogen? Women in estrogen dominance are likely to have PMS, too much body fat around the middle and difficulty losing weight. This particular hormone balance has also been shown to be the leading cause of breast, uterine, and prostate cancers.

Or, you may have low progesterone levels. Progesterone helps stimulate proper thyroid function in women, so when progesterone levels decrease due to a response to high levels of stress, the body "steals" progesterone to make the stress hormone cortisol, leaving excess estrogen! This is the primary way your body produces too much estrogen.

Bigger bellies (higher waist to hip ratio) are found in both thin and overweight women. Any menopausal woman will tell you that her body proportions have changed. So the best thing to do is eat less and exercise more, right? Wrong. Doing so increases your physiological stress and there is evidence that this makes fat body parts even fatter. **Calories matter, but hormones matter more.** When it comes to where fat is stored and how to combat it— and how to balance hormones—stress is the issue above all else.

So what can you do today about starting on a hormone-balancing program that in turn relieves stress? *I am glad you asked.* Any type of short, extreme, or continuous chronic dieting is a stressor to the body and you want to avoid stressful changes. Don't go too low carb, too low fat, or too low calorie. Subtle, gradual changes in your diet and exercise are best.

Do eat good sources of insoluble fiber which binds to excess estrogen. Good sources are non-GMO rice bran, corn bran, and the skins on fruits and vegetables. Eat raw nuts, especially Brazil nuts, which are high in selenium, and almonds. Sunflower seeds, and seeds in general, are a great source of insoluble fiber.

Did you know that the liver breaks down estrogen? If you have been told you have fatty liver, high cholesterol, or consume alcohol, know that this can cause excess estrogen and in turn excess weight due to the stress put on your liver. 1mg of folic acid and a B-complex vitamin can decrease the negative effects.

Guess what else affects estrogen levels? Bacteria imbalances in the gut compromise the proper elimination of estrogen in the body. To counteract this, you may want to include a probiotic daily, with at least 15 billion units. Store it in the fridge and take one or two, on an empty stomach. You also need sufficient intake of zinc, vitamin B6, and magnesium to break down estrogens.

When too much estrogen builds up, your body considers it a toxin and tries to release it the same way as any other toxin. Infrared sauna treatments are an excellent way to rid your body of toxins and excess estrogen. Removing excess estrogen is essential for health and to prevent many cancers.

Boost Your Weight Loss with These Tips

Get your Zs: Remember our old friend, a good night's sleep? Well, guess what? Without it, you're likely to have additional hormonal imbalances, which leads to weight gain. Sleep deprivation causes adrenal cortisol issues and metabolism issues, which both lead to weight gain. Make a choice to make sleep a priority. What's more important, late night TV or a hormonally balanced, flat tummy? Set your DVR to record that talk show and make sure you're in bed early. Let me tell you, Girlfriends, I understand that getting enough sleep can be tough. Between working, taking care of my family, visiting with friends, and any personal time I manage to carve out for myself, sleep can sneak its way to the bottom of my list. But it's so important, we must make it a priority, simplify your life so you can get to bed at a decent hour.

Work smarter, not harder: Many people think they need to ramp up their exercise and cut calories to lose weight, but that often leads your body to enter "starvation mode." In this mode, your body holds onto fat cells for dear life, making it even harder to burn them off. It may seem counterintuitive, but don't eat less and exercise more. A better approach is to eat less and exercise less. Or eat more and exercise more. This creates actual fat loss, encouraging both calorie reduction and hormone balance.

Prioritize simplicity, convenience, and order: With all the hormones floating around in our bodies that can potentially become imbalanced, weight loss is hard, isn't it? That's why ThyroSisters need to find ways to make it as easy as possible. Do you find it difficult to find time to exercise? Try a short, high intensity workout like Tabata. Named after Dr. Izumi Tabata, this is an exercise training method offering maximum benefit with the least amount of time. 20 seconds of all out exercise followed by 10 seconds of rest.

Don't have time to cook? Throw some vegetables, herbs, and chicken breasts into a slow cooker for a meal that greets you when you get home from work. Fill your shopping list with healthy fruits, veggies, and lean meats before you go to the grocery store, and only buy what's on the list. We all struggle with something different when it comes to weight loss. Brainstorm on your own or talk to your fellow ThyroSisters at www.ThyroSisters.com to come up with ways to streamline your health goals!

Take the right supplements: There are a few supplements that have been shown to help control the cortisol hypothalamus/

119

pituitary control center. The omega 3 fish oils, adaptogens (rhodiola ashwagandha, curcumin) are all helpful. Check your local natural foods market or drug store for these.

Hypochlorhydria

When the stomach doesn't produce enough stomach acid, a condition called hypochlorhydria is often the result. We need sufficient stomach acid to trigger the pancreas to release enzymes, and the gallbladder to release bile and cholecystokinin (one of the satiety hormones). Sufficient stomach acid also helps to establish healthy gut flora. "But Dr. Joni," you may be wondering, "if I'm trying to lose weight, who cares if I'm not digesting everything I eat?" Unfortunately, foods like carbs and sugars are easier to digest than other nutrients to include vitamins, minerals, and proteins. If food isn't digested properly, you don't absorb enough nutrients, and you'll crave even more food in an effort to get them.

Brain Chemistry

So far we've looked at a lot of ways in which different systems in the body heavily affect others, especially your big, brilliant brain. Well, guess what ladies? Hypothyroidism, food intolerances, inflammation, and hormonal imbalances are no different. They too tamper with the delicate balance of neurotransmitters in the brain.

Just like hormones govern many chemical functions in the body, messengers known as neurotransmitters govern the brain's chemical functions. T3 is the thyroid hormone that affects almost every physiological process in the body; temperature, heart rate, and metabolism. It's actually a neurotransmitter that regulates the action of serotonin, norepinephrine, and GABA (an inhibitory neurotransmitter that is important in reducing anxiety). Imbalances in these neurotransmitters tend to stimulate cravings, addictive behavior, anxiety, depression, and other disorders that often lead to overeating.

All the dietary protocols and nutritional compounds discussed in this book help restore balance to the brain and body. In order to turn your body into a fat-burning machine, all the systems have to work properly to burn fat for fuel, instead of storing it.

There are no quick or easy gimmicks to lasting weight loss. It's about addressing your overall health, especially the issues just discussed. The factors that cause one to be overweight can, of course, be complex and go beyond the physiological. Counseling, hypnotherapy, or a support group may be helpful to address emotional or subconscious components that contribute to being overweight. However, by improving the overall health of your body and brain, your losing battle with weight loss may soon be transformed into a victory.

Secrets Whispered to a ThyroSister

Although following a specific diet is the most important thing you can do to balance blood sugar and hormones, I find taking the right supplements can turbo-boost your results. Below is a list of the ingredients in the products I use in my practice for blood sugar problems:

- For hypoglycemia: Chromium, adrenal glandular, liver glandular, pancreas glandular, inositol, l-carnitine, CoQ10, rubidium, vanadium, and good quality, highly absorbable B vitamins.

- For insulin resistance: Chromium, alpha lipoic acid, N-acetylcysteine, l-carnitine, Poria Cocos, Gymnema sylvestre, Dioscerea, banana leaf, bitter melon, and nopal cactus.

- Go to www.ThyroSisters.com for up-to-date information about health issues that get in the way of effective weight loss.

- Increase the amount of healthy fiber in your diet.

- Increase your intake of water.

- Do a gut health panel, which can be done from the convenience of your home. We need to find the culprit causing your health imbalances, which could be parasites, mold, fungus, yeast, bacteria, or a virus. Visit www.ThyroSisters.com for more information about comprehensive lab testing.

- Read *Crazy, Sexy, Diet* by Kris Carr (10-year cancer survivor) about the benefits of eating a plant based diet, and the effects this lifestyle has on autoimmune diseases and cancer into remission. Also, try *Six Weeks to Sleeveless and Sexy* by JJ Virgin for great practical weight loss tips. Her new book, *The Virgin Diet: Drop 7 Foods, Lose 7 Pounds in 7 Days* details the most "offending foods" to which you may have a sensitivity.

CHAPTER 8
BUILD SMARTER:
Fix How Your Brain Functions

> " Are you still forgetting things?"
> 'I don't know,
> I can't remember,' I said. "
>
> *Stephen King*

Anna, 40, had no idea her brain was in trouble. Instead she came to see me for a sudden decline in her dental health: cavities, root canals, multiple gum grafts, and bleeding gums. She had also begun to suffer from hormonal difficulties, with periods coming closer together. When I questioned her specifically about brain symptoms, she confessed to experiencing memory loss and perpetual brain fog. "I walk into a room and forget why I went in there in the first place. And sometimes it's just so hard to concentrate at work. I never used to have these problems." Her mother and grandmother had experienced the same difficulties. "And now my grandmother has Alzheimer's disease! Is that going to happen to me, too?" She swallowed hard to hold back the tears.

"Let's see what we can do to avoid that," I said. I did a comprehensive panel of blood tests on Anna since most common brain disorders today stem from poor nutrition, digestive problems, low thyroid function, chronic inflammation, blood sugar imbalances, or chronic stress. I read the results of Anna's lab work differently than most medical doctors do. Typically doctors look for indications of diseases. I do that too, but I also look for trends toward disease.

For instance, a conventional doctor is likely to consider your thyroid functioning normal if lab results for thyroid stimulating hormone (TSH) fall within the range of 0.45 to 4.5 U/mL (units of TSH per milliliter of blood). I use a much narrower range of 1.8 to 3 U/mL, a standard that is used across the country in functional medicine. This more limited range allows me to detect a thyroid disorder in the early stages, and then address the common accompanying symptoms of depression, brain fog, and fatigue, using 'tools' from natural medicine to treat the condition before it becomes irreversible.

In order to treat Anna effectively, I also had her complete a neurotransmitter assessment form, designed by Dr. Kharrizan that asks questions designed to rate the performance of the brain. The form asks questions like, "Do you get sleepy after driving over an hour?" and "Are you more impatient than you used to be?" and "Can you easily count backwards from 100 in increments of 7?" From this extensive questionnaire we can gain a great understanding of how your brain's main neurotransmitters are working. Some of these neurotransmitters, chemicals that relay information, include serotonin, dopamine, GABA, and acetylcholine. For Anna, I also ran a urine/saliva kit that gave us detailed information on her neurotransmitter status, and also cortisol (the stress hormone) and the sex hormones progesterone, estrogen, and testosterone. These neurotransmitters can become imbalanced when health declines, causing mood disorders and numerous brain problems.

CONFESSIONS OF A GLUTEN-FREE CONVERT

Kathy, a 57-year-old attractive professional came into my office looking for answers to headaches, hormone imbalances, and fatigue. She thought she was doing everything "right" for these issues to include taking bio-identical hormones, exercising, and eating well. This is what she had to say about her experience and what finally worked:

When Dr. Labbe suggested that I go on a gluten-free diet I was skeptical, to say the least. How could this possibly help? I wondered. But since I was suffering from painful migraines that were getting worse, and freaked out by the aura that I experienced every time, and since the prescription offered by my neurologist was making things worse, I was willing to try anything.

So out of desperation, and perhaps to show her how wrong she was, I decided to give this gluten-free thing a whirl for a few days, I never expected it to work...

But here's the deal, I haven't had a migraine, or an aura, or even a bad headache, since going gluten-free. Yet this stunning fact is just the beginning of the changes that happened in my body as a result. The way I understand this now, I was poisoning myself every time I ate, so when I stopped doing so the results were quite dramatic.

I lost weight simply by making different food choices. The abdominal bloating went away, as did my cravings for sugar, especially chocolate. The internal trembling I'd put up with for years disappeared. After a few weeks I noticed feeling nourished and happy after eating reasonable amounts of healthy foods, and I started to crave them; no I couldn't believe it either. The brain fog I'd accepted as a part of aging also dissipated.

A gluten-free lifestyle was surely not the solution I had envisioned in dealing with the curse of debilitating migraines, but it has been a solution I can live with!

A Gluten-Free Diet for Better Brain Health

The effects of gluten on brain health are beautifully documented in David Perlmutter's excellent book, *Grain Brain*. However, Anna learned all about it first hand, as her results showed that she had gluten and dairy intolerances, so I advised her to eat a strict gluten-free and dairy-free diet. While the diet was strict, the new sense of freedom and well-being was empowering for Anna. After three months on the new diet and supplements to include phosphatidylserine, SAMe, folic acid, fish oil, l-tryptophan (for memory, depression, and anxiety), Anna's dental and hormonal symptoms cleared, and her brain fog lifted. She felt more alert and energetic, her memory returned, concentration improved, and she felt better equipped to handle the stress in her life.

However, the importance of her new diet didn't sink in completely until Anna ate gluten during a vacation and her symptoms returned with a merciless vengeance. Her gums began bleeding again, she became severely constipated, her motivation tanked, and the menstrual irregularities returned. After that slip-up, Anna is careful to stick to her gluten and dairy-free diet in order to enjoy her life without experiencing any frustrating or debilitating symptoms.

When Hormones Decline

When we think of hormone troubles we usually think of the uterus and ovaries, bleeding or not bleeding, and sex hormones. **The truth is the most important reproductive organ in our body is the brain.** The reason perimenopause and menopause can be so awful is largely because of the impact fluctuating or declining hormones have on the brain. Estrogen in particular is vital to the female brain, and when levels start to decline, the brain loses a chemical that helped create it, and has kept it running effectively for years. Not surprisingly, symptoms like brain fog, memory loss, and loss of fine motor control (such as being able to do embroidery or other work with the fingers) kick in when estrogen levels decline. This estrogen decline is due to the ovaries gradually producing less estrogen as you move into menopause. Estrogen is crucial for thinking and remembering. Problems with mood, sleep, anxiety, and depression are also often related to declining levels of estrogen in the brain.

Women are also more vulnerable to assaults on the brain, through injury or emotional distress, when estrogen is low. An estrogen-deprived brain will sustain more damage from a head injury, for example, or leave a woman more vulnerable to anxiety, depression, or post-traumatic stress disorder (PTSD). Until recently, researchers had largely dismissed the influences of female hormones on the brain and mental health. Fortunately, this is now changing and more information is becoming available.

It's important to manage your hormones during the menopausal transition so you feel better and are more resilient in the event of an injury or trauma. Car accidents, falls, mountain bike crashes…stuff happens. Estrogen plays an important role in both protecting your brain, and recovering, from physical and emotional trauma.

If you are in the throes of menopause, you usually have low estrogen. Estrogen directly affects brain function through estrogen receptors located in multiple areas of the brain (Birge, HRT and Cognition: What the Evidence Shows, 2000). Estrogen has been shown to protect isolated neurons from numerous forms of damage (McKeun BS, 1999), including:

- **Oxidative stress:** the available supply of the body's antioxidants is insufficient to handle and neutralize free radicals, causing massive cell damage.

- **Ischemic injury:** insufficient blood flow to the brain to meet metabolic demand leads to poor oxygen supply.

- **Hypoglycemic injury:** low glucose commonly causes brain fuel deprivation.

- **Damage by amyloid protein:** which is implicated in Alzheimer's disease.

Estrogen also stimulates production of nerve growth factors, promoting nerve growth, repair of damaged neurons, and dendritic branching (Birge, 1997).

As you can see, the environment of low estrogen levels and trauma sets up a downward cascade of inflammation, decreased anti-oxidants, insufficient blood supply, and damaged nerve growth. This situation would make it harder to make a comeback from trauma, emotional or physical.

If that wasn't enough, low estrogen levels may also be responsible for one of the most well-known parts of menopause. Hot flashes are a classic symptom of menopause, a sudden sensation of heat in the upper body, often followed by perspiration and chills. Heart racing and sweating have been documented to occur during a hot flash. Although poorly understood, these episodes originate in the brain, most likely as a direct response to low estrogen in the hypothalamus (RR Freedman, 1990). Additionally, it appears that hot flashes lead to other neurological problems. Hot flashes have been directly correlated to memory impairment.

What You Eat Impacts the Health of Your Brain

Lack of estrogen isn't the only thing wreaking havoc in our brains. The modern American diet, with its high sugar content and overabundance of processed ingredients, is devastating the brains of many Americans (I'll talk more about this later). The proof is in the numbers; the US leads the world in the prevalence of mood and mental disorders, which currently affect one in four Americans (Kessler RC, 2005). And the number of people suffering from depression, anxiety, insomnia, mental illness, substance abuse, Alzheimer's disease, and Parkinson's disease is rising.

Adults aren't the only ones negatively affected. The rates of childhood autism, attention deficit hyperactivity disorder (ADHD), obsessive-compulsive disorder (OCD), Tourette's syndrome, and learning disabilities (such as dyslexia) have exploded (Rice, 2009), (Baio, 2012). New research shows that poor parental health affects brain development in utero and after a child is born, creating tendencies toward autism spectrum disorders, ADHD, and learning disabilities (Hertz-Picciotto I, 2006). If poor nutrition is affecting a woman's health, it will affect the health of her unborn children as well.

Feeding the Brain

Your brain uses 20 percent of your energy, even though it comprises only two percent of your weight. Eating to support your brain health helps you retain your memory, maintain a good mood, and stay sharp into old age. Antioxidants and essential fatty acids (EFAs) help preserve brain tissue, reduce inflammation, and support the ability of the neurons to build new communication pathways. Water is also important, since it makes up over 70% of the brain (Perlman, 2014). So is fat, which is why healthy, natural fats (such as raw nuts, avocadoes, and salmon) are a critically important part of a healthy diet.

What does not support the health of the brain is consuming sugars and starchy foods, processed vegetable oils, hydrogenated fats, or chemical additives. Food intolerances wreak havoc in the body, and the brain too. High-carb diets are now being linked to serious neurological disorders such as Alzheimer's disease, Parkinson's disease, and multiple sclerosis (Perlmutter, 2013).

But here's the good news. **The brain thrives when it's nourished with EFAs** (essential fatty acids), particularly eicosapentaenoic acid (EPA) and docosahexaenoic acid (DHA), both found naturally in omega 3 fatty acids. DHA is the most abundant fat in the brain, and is plentiful in cold-water fish such as wild salmon, mackerel, halibut, scallops, sardines, and herring. Vegetarian sources of these essential fatty acids are flax, walnuts, and in lesser amounts, black currant, pumpkin, and other seeds and seed oils.

To utilize healthy fats, your body must convert these sources to EPA and DHA, a process that can be impaired in people who have blood sugar disorders, or consume too many omega 6 fatty acids, such as palm, soybean, and sunflower oils.

Your brain also needs these vitamins to maintain healthy functioning:

- **Thiamine** helps metabolize glucose, which the brain needs for energy. Foods rich in thiamine include trout, lean pork, macadamia nuts, sunflower seeds, and green peas.

- **B12** is needed to maintain the sheaths surrounding the nerves that facilitate communication between neurons, and helps prevent nerve damage and impaired brain function. Eat shellfish like clams and crab, red meat, Swiss cheese, and eggs.

- **Folate** helps to prevent depression and maintain cognitive function. To get enough, eat dark leafy greens like spinach, mustard greens, turnip greens, parsley, and collard greens. Beets, lentils, and cauliflower are great sources of folate, too.

- **B6** is essential to producing the brain's chemicals, called neurotransmitters. It also prevents depression, improves memory, and prevents dementia. Try bananas, avocados, salmon, chicken breast, sunflower seeds, and Brussels sprouts.

- **Antioxidants** to include Vitamin C and vitamin E help protect the brain from damage. Vitamin C is found in citrus fruits, strawberries, kale, broccoli, guava, tomatoes, and peas. Tofu, spinach, almonds, avocados, and olive oil have high amounts of vitamin E.

Healthy Gut, Healthy Brain

Science is discovering that gut health profoundly affects brain health. In fact, researchers have discovered a link between depression (and other mental disorders) and gut inflammation (Bested AC, 2013). Bloating, gas, pain, heartburn, diarrhea, constipation, and food sensitivities may seem like inconveniences; after all, you see commercials for gut remedies all the time. But these are not harmless symptoms; in fact they're big red flags that your body is waving to get your attention. These are strong signals that your brain is under attack.

Who are the attackers? Commonly, it's your very own immune system, armed with a double-edged sword: inflammation. There are different ways your brain can become inflamed, but one of the main ways doesn't even start in your brain; it starts in your "second brain," the gut. And you would never even know it. Just like your brain, the inner mucosal lining of your gut has no pain fibers, so even though health issues may start in your gut, it won't tell you there's a problem.

So how does your gut inflame your brain? It all starts with a protein called Zonulin. I know, zonu-what? Zonulin is a cytokine, or immune system protein, that's released during inflammatory gut conditions like leaky gut. Due to intestinal bacteria, overgrowth of yeast, or parasitic infection, it opens up the intestinal tight junctions that form the barrier between your digestive system and the rest of your body. Zonulin, along with other toxins, then starts to circulate freely throughout your body, causing, you guessed it, systemic inflammation. And not only can Zonulin open up your protective gut lining, it can also open your protective blood-brain barrier, too, leading the charge for toxins entering your brain (Fasano, 2001). Leaky gut equals leaky brain!

Toxins escaping from your intestines aren't the only problem. A primary nerve connects the brain and the digestive system (the vagus nerve), so communication between the gut and brain is direct and intimate, like two best friends who spend all day texting. If you have a friend like that, then you know how confusing it is if she suddenly stops answering your texts, right?

About fifty percent of your brain is made up of glia cells; immune cells that turn on an inflammatory response in your brain. This chronic inflammation can decrease neuron firing, causing decreased communication with the gut, impairing the gut's function and causing even more inflammation that starts a downward spiral (Dantzer R, 2008). From all this inflammation, it's just a short hop, skip, and a jump to sickness and depression, as the immune system subjugates the brain with inflammation. Brain inflammation can also impact your communication with the rest of your body via the hormone system, such as the thyroid, and the adrenal glands,(Psychiatr Pol. 2002;36(2):281-92) leaving you tired, brain fogged, cranky and overweight.

So, the moral of the story is this: **what affects the brain eventually affects the gut**, which explains why people with head injuries, dementia, or autism often have gut problems. What affects the gut also affects the brain, so one of the best ways to shore up your brain health is to mend your gut.

Lifting the Brain Fog

One of the most common complaints I hear from patients is the experience of having 'brain fog', the feeling that a thick, lingering fog shrouds the brain. Thinking is slow, and there's a sense that one's body is detached from the world, or tuned into a different channel than everyone else.

As Dr. Kharrazian explains in his book *Why Isn't My Brain Working?*, brain fog is the result of brain inflammation that slows conductivity between the neurons in the brain. It's like your neurons have to walk through sand to send messages. Inflammation in your knee or elbow causes pain, but the brain does not have pain fibers. Brain inflammation and brain fog are very common in clients whose autoimmune Hashimoto's hypothyroidism is not well managed. Some people experience brain fog when they eat food they are allergic to, are exposed to toxic chemicals, or suffer from sleep deprivation, blood sugar imbalances, or a head injury. Women going through menopause often complain of brain fog, because declining and fluctuating estrogen inflames their brain.

Brain fog is a warning that your brain health is compromised and you need to take action to improve your health. For most people this means following the earlier recommendations on restoring gut and adrenal health. If you are suffering from multiple symptoms of hormone deficiency and unable to restore hormonal balance, you may need bioidentical hormone replacement therapy to protect your brain. It's also recommended to follow basic functional medicine principles to improve your overall health.

Even with doing all we've discussed, there are times when you may need some supplemental support to reduce chronic brain inflammation and clear the brain fog. I use a formula of botanicals that quench brain inflammation and reduce or remove brain fog. The formula includes catechins (a type of antioxidant) from green tea extract, curcumin, rutin, baicalin, resveratrol, apigenin, and luteolin.

Seven common culprits that may be causing your brain fog

1. Hormone changes, especially low estrogen levels
2. Poor diet, including too much sugar or carbohydrates
3. Low consumption of essential fatty acids
4. Undiagnosed or untreated gut issues
5. Inflammation in the brain
6. Imbalanced neurotransmitters
7. Poor blood flow to the brain

Can Your Brain Breathe?

Poor blood flow to the brain means the brain is not getting enough oxygen, and this is another common cause of brain fog. The blood carries oxygen, which allows the brain to breathe. Just like an athlete can't run far without oxygen, your brain can't function at its peak without this vital fuel. If your fingers and toes are always cold, if your nose is cold, if you are prone to chronic nail fungus, if you suffer from anemia, or smoke, the circulation in your brain may be impaired. Cold extremities are a strong sign blood is not reaching the outermost parts of the body. Unfortunately, this includes the brain. If you don't have enough oxygen available to supply your brain and nervous system, then other treatments may not be effective.

Managing Hashimoto's hypothyroidism, anemia, and other health issues will improve blood flow to the brain. I use a formula to support blood flow in the brain that includes magnesium citrate, feverfew, Butcher's Broom, Ginkgo biloba, cayenne pepper, and vinpocetine. These herbs can be found through your health care professional, or at health food stores.

Balancing Brain Chemicals
- Four Critical Brain Neurotransmitters
- Serotonin
- GABA
- Dopamine
- Acetvlcholine

Sometimes even when you're doing all the right things, your brain chemicals (neurotransmitters), may still be a bit off. Fluctuations in hormones, stress levels, and other life factors can disrupt this important balance. Since the nervous system runs the show, it controls virtually all of the body's responses to daily stimuli, such as heart rate, digestion, sleep and metabolism. To control these functions, the nervous system sends and receives information from the brain to every single cell. Neurotransmitters are the chemicals that carry the nervous system's messages to and from the rest of the body; they give the body's various systems a way to communicate with each other.

In order to make sure your nervous system is sending the right signals, it's important to test neurotransmitter levels. Neurotransmitter test results are like biochemical fingerprints; each one is unique and provides a wealth of clinical information. Urinary neurotransmitters are peripheral measurements, but act as biomarkers for the central and peripheral nervous system activity. Urinary test results cannot diagnose neurotransmitter imbalances, but they can give valuable information about how the body is functioning.

Neurotransmitters excreted in the urine can be viewed as biomarkers to provide insight into nervous system function, and reveal many clinical conditions. You can order test collection materials, with information about specimen collection, paperwork completion, insurance, and the return of your specimens to the lab, at www.ThyroSisters.com. Look for Pharmasan Labs test kits.

Neurotransmitter imbalances can be correlated with a wide variety of health conditions such as depression, sleep difficulties, fatigue, anxiety, and behavior disorders. Providing support for the neurotransmitters can profoundly improve your mood, sense of well-being, and brain function. There are several ways to balance neurotransmitters so that your perception of life is calm, optimistic, and filled with vibrancy. An increased understanding of the neurotransmitters in your brain will help you identify what may be causing your brain fog and other brain related issues, as well as what you can do about it.

• *Serotonin: The joy and well-being neurotransmitter*

This neurotransmitter delivers a sense of well-being, prevents depression, and ensures a good night's sleep. If you're approaching or going through menopause, it's especially important to know about serotonin, because it is profoundly influenced by estrogen. When estrogen levels fall, serotonin levels do too, frequently leaving you with a bad case of the blues. Serotonin is also a precursor to melatonin, an important sleep hormone, so adequate levels of serotonin are needed in order to sleep well at night.

Blood sugar imbalances impair serotonin activity as well. If you struggle with hypoglycemia or insulin resistance, you need to be aware of the impact of these imbalances on your serotonin levels.

Symptoms of low serotonin:
- Feelings of constant depression or sadness
- Fatigue, even when you sleep well
- Sleep disturbances
- Lack of interest in things that used to be enjoyable
- Cravings for sweets and starches
- Low self-esteem
- Mood worsens due to lack of light

If better nutrition and improved blood sugar balance, adrenal health, and gut repair fail to alleviate symptoms of low serotonin, certain amino acids and botanicals will improve your serotonin status. Start with the recommended dose, and gradually increase your dose each time you take it, until you begin to notice improvement.

Nutrients to support serotonin. These include St. John's Wort, SAMe, and 5-HTP. For those who cannot tolerate 5-HTP products I recommend L-tryptophan, which supports serotonin in a more gradual dose-responsive curve. L-Theanine has been widely studied for its ability to produce calming effects.

• *Acetylcholine: The learning and memory neurotransmitter*

Acetylcholine is a neurotransmitter that deserves close attention during menopause, since learning and memory tend to go south, along with estrogen, for many women during this transition. Symptoms of low acetylcholine often look like memory loss and dementia, so if you feel like your ability to remember things is slipping, you will want to support this neurotransmitter. Healthy acetylcholine levels depend on good dietary fats; therefore people on ultra low-fat diets may have impaired acetylcholine activity.

Symptoms of low acetylcholine:
- Memory loss or lapses
- Poor visual memory
- Reduced creativity
- Diminished ability to calculate numbers (For example the ability to count backwards in increments of 7)
- Slow to process and respond
- Difficulty with spatial orientation or directions

Nutrients to support acetylcholine. These include pantothenic acid, alpha-GPC, N-acetyl L-carnitine, and huperzine A.

• *GABA: The calm and relaxed neurotransmitter*

Gamma aminobutyric acid (GABA) is the anti-anxiety chemical responsible for keeping the brain calm and tranquil. As with the other neurotransmitters, poor diet, poor overall health, and blood sugar imbalances can contribute to low GABA function. Gluten intolerance may deplete GABA levels by causing an autoimmune attack against the enzyme that makes it; this is actually more common than most people realize. If you suffer from chronic anxiety, a gluten-free diet should be first on your list of ways to significantly improve your health.

Some people have a genetic inability to make enough GABA. When this happens the enzyme that triggers the production of GABA is impaired, and these people suffer from some degree of anxiety throughout their lives. Taking supplements regularly to encourage GABA production could help you cope better with life's challenges, including menopause, or your 16-year-old son getting his driver's license!

Symptoms of low GABA activity include:
- Feelings of panic, dread, or anxiety
- Inner tension, butterflies, or knot in the stomach
- Restless mind, can't relax
- Feeling overwhelmed for no real reason
- Lack of focus, disorganized, poor attention
- Frequent, constant worrying

Nutrients to support GABA. You cannot get GABA from the foods you eat, but some contain the building block for this neurotransmitter, the amino acid l-glutamine. Pork, beef, sesame and sunflower seeds contain glutamine. You may need to take supplemental GABA on an as-needed basis (such as to improve sleep), or for a short period of time while you get other health issues in order. I use cutting edge GABA compounds that include L-taurine, valerian root, passion flower, L-theanine, lithium, 4-amino-3-phenylbutyric acid (a GABA agonist), and B6, an important cofactor for the synthesis of GABA.

• *Dopamine: The pleasure and reward neurotransmitter*

Dopamine allows us to feel pleasure and a sense of reward. It is most commonly associated with addiction because habit-forming substances, or activities, activate this neurotransmitter. Every time you gamble, take a puff from a cigarette, or binge eat, your brain releases dopamine. Dopamine's allure is so powerful that when rats are given a choice between a shot of dopamine or food and water, they will continually choose dopamine – until they die from starvation and dehydration (Gutierrez, 2010).

Low dopamine levels are associated with feelings of low self-worth, bouts of rage, and lack of drive or motivation. (If this sounds like your husband, it's because low testosterone levels lead to diminished dopamine.) Dopamine is also associated with progesterone, so if your progesterone level is low, you may be suffering from symptoms of inadequate dopamine as well.

Symptoms of low dopamine:
- Lack of drive or motivation, difficulty finishing tasks
- Feelings of worthlessness or hopelessness
- Easily lose your temper
- Feeling angry and aggressive when stressed
- Isolating yourself from others, wanting to "hole up"
- Lack of concern for, or sense of detachment from, loved ones

Nutrients to support dopamine. A number of vegetables are excellent sources of the amino acids that stimulate dopamine production. For example, beets contain the amino acid betaine, which aids in the regulation of dopamine. Artichokes, avocados, strawberries, blueberries, and prunes are full of nutrients that trigger the release of dopamine. If diet and lifestyle changes fail to correct low levels of dopamine, I have gotten great results using supplements that contain Mucuna pruriens, DL-phenylalanine, beta-phenylethylamine, N-acetyl L-tyrosine, N-acetyl L-cysteine, blueberry extract, and alpha lipoic acid.

When You Need Advanced Brain Support

Some brain imbalances have been hardwired since birth, or are the result of trauma or injury to the brain. In these situations a person needs more than diet or supplements can deliver. Direct brain activation exercises may be the solution. Practitioners of functional neurology can often help with seemingly irresolvable brain, gut, or other health issues; Frederick Carrick, DC, PhD, a world-renowned neurologist developed many of these principles.

The therapies he suggests for brain activation include vibration therapy, simple balance exercises, auditory (sound) stimulation in one ear, auricular stimulation (acupressure of ear points), warm calorics in one ear (warm water infusions in one ear to fire up the hemisphere of the brain that is not firing as readily), and visual stimulation of one eye. These treatments help to correct the brain's misfiring and positively influence the production of cortisol and other hormones, blood sugar regulation, oxygen deficits, and other health issues. While these treatments may not be a popular part of mainstream medicine, I've had great success using them to help kick start some clients' brains.

Functional neurologists have discovered that brain imbalances, brain inflammation, and brain degeneration are the cause of many aging-related symptoms such as incontinence, high blood pressure, dry eyes, poor balance, light sensitivity, and headaches (Chopdar A, 2003), (Griffiths DJ, 2009), (Benarroch, 2007). The brain governs all of these functions, but sometimes areas of the brain don't fire, or transmit signals properly (either firing too much or too little). This causes nerves, vessels, and other areas of the brain to function improperly. Perhaps you have been "worked up" by a traditional neurologist and given a prescription for the neurological complaint. Maybe there was a positive effect for a while, and then the problems returned.

When confronted with chronic pain, deterioration of autonomic (bodily) functions, memory loss, or other symptoms of brain degeneration, it's important to have a comprehensive functional neurological and metabolic evaluation. If you have experienced a head trauma, or suffer from lifelong imbalances related to ADHD, autism, dyslexia, or other learning disabilities; if you feel your brain is aging too quickly, or if you suffer from deterioration of autonomic function or poor balance, you are likely to benefit from all that functional neurology has to offer.

Brain Autoimmunity

Another condition I often see in clients with brain disorders is autoimmunity to their brain tissue. You read this correctly; this is a condition in which the immune system mistakenly attacks and destroys its own brain tissue. Autoimmune reactions in the brain, and against nervous tissue, are not uncommon and it's important in many cases to test for brain autoimmunity.

Fibromyalgia: It Sort of is "All in Your Head"

Fibromyalgia is a crippling disease that is currently ruining the lives of over 10 million people. Nearly nine out of ten are women (National Fibromyalia Association, 2009). Melody, 42, came to me anxious about her health. "I just came back from the doctor, and I matched a fibromyalgia questionnaire." Her voice trembled a bit as she spoke. "I have pain in my joints and in all the places that a fibromyalgia patient has. Yet my friends and other people say there is no such thing as fibromyalgia, that I just need anti-depressants or anti-anxiety medication."

Well, that's simply not true. Fibromyalgia and the pain it causes are very real. What many people do not know, or understand, is that fibromyalgia is a neurological condition. This explanation gets a bit technical, but hang with me, because if you suffer from this disorder you need to understand this. Fibromyalgia is a signal that brain health is compromised, that in fact your brain is aging too quickly. The longer you have fibromyalgia the more quickly your brain ages, which is a nice way of saying that brain cells are dying.

There are three parts to your brainstem: top (mesencephalon), middle (pons), and bottom (medulla). Normally the brain fires impulses down to the lower two parts of the brainstem, and that slows down the upper brainstem. With a fibromyalgia patient, this important process in the brain is not happening. The lower part of the brainstem is not slowing down the upper brainstem which causes urinary tract infections, sensitivity to light, insomnia, increased heart rate, pain, and fatigue. (Dr. Michael Johnson, author of *What Do You Do When the Medications Don't Work*).

So what causes the physical pain associated with this disorder? When the upper brainstem is over firing, it drives down an area of the spinal cord called the IML (intermediolateral) cell nucleus, which causes the adrenal glands to release stress hormones that stimulate the smallest and most painful fibers, and the pain fibers become over stimulated, specifically Type C pain fibers. The latest research points to brainstem injury, or malfunction, as a major cause of fibromyalgia, pain, dizziness, headaches, and insomnia (Fallon N, 2013), (Jasmin, 2012), (Goadsby, 2002), (Duning T, 2013).

Other common and frustrating conditions have a neurological explanation and can be successfully addressed through functional neurology and functional medicine.

- **Irritable Bowel Syndrome (IBS):** This condition is characterized by episodes of diarrhea, constipation, abdominal pain, nausea, and even vomiting. Experts don't completely understand what causes IBS. Some theories say it is a problem with bowel motility; the muscles in the bowels don't contract normally, causing constipation. Other studies suggest the colon is hypersensitive, going into spasms. Instead of slow, rhythmic muscle contractions the bowel muscles spasm, causing diarrhea or constipation. Another theory suggests that the nerve signals that regulate communication between the gut and the brain, may be involved. An area in the lower brainstem called NTS (nucleus tractus solitarius) is the origin of the vagus nerve that carries impulses directly to your abdomen. So if you are suffering with IBS, constipation or Crohn's disease, your lower brainstem may not be transmitting the way that it should.

- **Headaches:** You may have headaches because your brain is not firing impulses to the lower brainstem, and the lower brainstem is supposed to slow down the upper brainstem. In headache sufferers, this system is not firing correctly. Sometimes in the case of a migraine sufferer, this causes light sensitivity because the pupil fails to constrict due to decreased firing of the third cranial nerve.

- **Brain Fog:** Decreased firing of neurons in the frontal and temporal lobes of the brain is often responsible for brain fog. If you have difficulty expressing what you want to say, the dysfunction is in the area of the brain called Broca's speech area, in the left frontal lobe (the area of the forehead). This also causes an increased heart rate, due to the upper brainstem over firing.

- **Dizziness:** Near the back of the brain is an area called the cerebellum. Many clients complain to me that they have problems with brain fog, difficulty putting thoughts into words, or dizziness. Since the cerebellum controls all your spinal muscles, it affects balance and coordination. When a person with fibromyalgia is dizzy or lightheaded, firing from the cerebellum has slowed.

It's important to keep in mind when dealing with the health of your brain that you are NOT crazy, lazy, or finished, and most likely you are not losing your mind either, even if you can't remember where you put your keys. Get to the root cause of your brain related symptoms by using the principles, ideas and suggestions in this book.

A "Prescription" For Supplements

I have great success with using a variety of scientifically chosen supplements to help women regain their mojo by addressing the source of their symptoms. Adding this support to your daily routine may seem a bit overwhelming at first, until you get used to doing so and start to experience improvement.

In most cases it's a good idea to start adding supplements slowly, paying close attention to how your body reacts, and then increasing the amount when your body begins to get used to the ingredients. (Keep in mind that once your health issues are successfully identified and treated, you may be able to reduce or stop the supplementation.) It's always important to let the health professional you're working with know how your body is reacting to your new protocol, to include improvements and any concerns.

By the way, you can use the 'placebo effect' to your advantage in adding supplements to your health protocol. If you start taking them with the conviction that this is exactly what your body needs and has been 'asking for' you enhance your opportunity to get great results!

- Check out Pharmason Labs. This is an excellent lab with accurate tests to measure nervous, endocrine, and immune system markers, using an easy, at home urine test.

- In cases where autoimmunity to brain tissue is suspected, get an antibody panel against neurological tissue from Cyrex Labs. A link to this labs may be found at www.ThyroSisters.com

- Repair leaky gut. If this is an issue for you, it will make a significant difference in your health and decrease inflammation in your body and brain.

- Spectra-Cell Laboratories Inc. is a specialized clinical testing laboratory company. They specialize in micro-nutrient testing, nutritional deficiencies, cardio-metabolic testing.

- Genova Diagnostics is a global leader in functional laboratory testing. They offer innovative laboratory assessments in endocrine assessments, nutrition, genomics, and digestive health.

- ZRT Laboratory uses cutting-edge technology to deliver convenient, minimally invasive saliva testing and blood spot testing services.

CHAPTER 9
BUILDING YOU UP:
How to Maintain an Active Attitude

If you want a good knock to the head, tell a woman in the throes of menopausal symptoms to "think positive." When you are suffering deeply from pain, anxiety, depression, insomnia, hot flashes, or other serious health problems, being told to develop a positive attitude feels like a belittling brush off. Often it's a way for people to ignore you, bury their head in denial, or think they are helping you.

But there is a great secret I want to share with you. Earl Nightingale called it, "the strangest secret in the world." This secret is so powerful that it has changed the lives of millions of people. I am referring to the secret Mr. Nightingale elaborated on almost fifty years ago when he stated, *"What you think about the most is what you eventually become."*

What he was teaching in making this statement is that what you allow to control your daily thoughts will serve as a magnet that will pull similar thoughts and circumstances to it, whether you consciously want to do so or not. This is an inspiring truth that has been around for ages. Albert Einstein once said, "Imagination is

146

everything. It is the preview of life's coming attractions." In Proverbs 23:7 it says, *"As a man thinketh in his heart, so is he."*

While telling someone in pain to "think positive" may be initially perceived poorly, **the truth is that thinking positively, concentrating on the good in your life, and re-framing your perspective can profoundly influence your health**, and the success of your efforts to heal. But you don't have to go around pretending you're happy when you're really not. If you're in the throes of suffering and feel miserable, look at adopting a positive approach to healing like an exercise plan or brushing your teeth, something important you do every day for a short period of time.

Research has demonstrated that committing to even a few minutes of optimistic thoughts once or twice a day, produces measurable benefits (Scheier MF, 1993). Just as you build muscle with physical exercise, regular positive thinking exercises build new pathways in your brain that lead you to feel better and view your situation in more positive terms. Over time your healing mojo will gather momentum, and you will gradually grow happier and more optimistic, which profoundly impacts your immune system, ability to handle stress, your digestive system, hormone balance, and many other aspects of health.

Positive Thinking Helps You Cope Better

I have to be honest with you, at this point the research regarding the effects of positive thinking on healing or curing an illness is mixed. Some studies show no correlation between positive thinking and health outcomes, such as in the case of cancer survival rates (Crompton, 2012). But the research suggests that while positive thinking can't guarantee a cure, it does help you cope better with your illness which could lead to sticking with your treatment plan and protocols (Scheier MF M. K., 1989). Over time this will help you get better.

The research does show that people with a chronic disease who think of something each morning that makes them feel good and who use self-affirmation techniques, like prayer or meditation when encountering obstacles, are consistently more compliant in following their treatment plan. Studies also show that patients with a positive spiritual belief system experience less depression and are better able to handle their medical situation (Pressman P, 1990).

In the book *Positivity,* author Barbara Fredrickson explains how building a habit of positivity makes you more resilient to the setbacks and hardships in life. Regularly focusing on joy, hope, amusement, gratitude, appreciation, awe, and other buoyant emotions lowers blood pressure and stress, and boosts expanded, creative thinking. Fredrickson has found that if your positive thoughts outnumber your negative thoughts by three to one, you can successfully combat feelings of negativity.

What are you cultivating in the fertile soil of your mind? Make a decision today to cultivate seeds of greatness, because that is what we are all intended to become. Do not allow anything else to dominate your thoughts. Begin to embrace this habit and your life will likely improve. The positive thoughts can be small; frequency is the key. **Both appreciation and gratitude are quick and easy emotions with large net effects.** You don't need to meet the three-to-one ratio every single time a negative emotion pops up—just make regular deposits into your positivity bank account to receive daily dividends.

Start Using "Possibilities Thinking"

Read the next sentence very carefully because it may just change your life. As my friend and colleague Dr. Louis Arrizo says, *"Nothing in this world is impossible until you tell yourself it is."* Think about it, this is so true!

Check your own inner voice. Have you been telling yourself, "This is impossible?" Staying focused on possibilities does not mean you will realize your goal in the time frame you'd like or that it will be easy. It doesn't mean you are going to enjoy every single second of the journey. Yet anything is possible and it's important to keep this in mind. Perhaps you just need to make an internal clarification: *what is the price you are willing to pay for the end result you desire?* We must all sacrifice something to learn, grow and achieve; this is a universal law. Do you want to choose what you are willing to make sacrifices to achieve, or do you want life to choose for you?

I recommend you make the choice consciously, because you may not appreciate what life deals you in its never-ending attempt to wake you up to your full potential. Possibilities thinking! What an awesome outlook on life. Are you willing to make changes in your diet? To cut out the sugar, gluten, or other foods your body is reacting to? Are you ready to take the necessary lab tests to clarify what's causing your health issues? Have you embraced the wisdom of lifestyle changes to include increased exercise, fresh air, clean water, and changing your "stinkin thinkin"?

ThyroSisters, your approach in improving your health and sense of well-being is completely up to you, but my recommendation is that it's well worth your time to pay close attention to your thoughts, and upgrade your belief in getting positive results.

You no longer have to accept having the blues or dragging yourself around as the norm. Your new upgraded belief system knows that while you're not perfect, you're sure heading in the right direction. We are not looking for perfection here, just progression. Through meditation, prayer, supplements, clean air, water, food, and friends, you will overcome these chronic health issues that have been plaguing you.

What is Stinkin' Thinkin'?

This term originally came out of the Alcoholics Anonymous (AA) recovery program, used to describe the denial of the addict who doesn't think he has a disease. It has since been widely embraced to describe the many ways our negative thoughts undermine our sense of well-being.

Internal negative thoughts such as: "I've lost my mojo and it's never coming back," work against our physical, mental, and spiritual health instead of supporting our efforts to feel good and move forward. What we think, even if we don't say it out loud, profoundly impacts what we do and how we feel. By unlearning and working to reverse our stinkin' thinkin' we increase our ability to heal, grow, learn, and get the positive results we deserve.

The Power of Physical Activity

Dr. Kharrazian jokes that if people had to run or walk to pick up their prescription for antidepressants, the rates of depression in our society would be much lower. The human body was designed to move and depriving it of movement is like depriving it of sunlight or social contact. Being sedentary might not kill you in the same way as going without air or water will, but it can sure kill your mood.

Numerous studies have linked exercise with significantly reduced rates of serious illnesses to include Alzheimer's, heart disease, cancer, stroke, diabetes, obesity, and high blood pressure (Brwon WJ, 2007), (Lytle ME, 2004). Consistent exercise also has been shown to alleviate depression and anxiety, and to improve mood. In a study of older people, regular exercise helped women eliminate symptoms of anxiety and depression associated with aging (Villaverde CG, 2012). It appears this is accomplished through the release of feel-good chemicals in the brain that reduce inflammation and raise core body temperature.

Changes in core body temperature are associated with significant changes in metabolic rate, raising the interesting possibility that differences in core temperature may play an important role in obesity and weight loss. **Let's face it ThyroSisters; when we look better, we feel better.** People who exercise regularly find that doing so improves confidence, relieves worry, helps with weight loss, balances hormones, improves sleep, and reduces stress.

Of course I know that finding the time or motivation to exercise can be challenging, especially when you are feeling lousy or beyond lousy. If your health is important to you, make it a point to place exercise at the top of your daily to-do list, and then slowly start adding more movement into your life. The good news is that once you push through the initial part where it feels like a major chore, the motivation will come more naturally as you begin to reap the benefits. The "exercise high" is real and very addictive, but this is one addiction you can indulge! (Providing you do not over exercise, which can cause adrenal fatigue or physical injury.)

Experiment at first until you identify the type of exercise that feels so good that you get hooked. Adding exercise to your life doesn't have to be grueling. Make it fun! Be creative; try varying your walking pace, how long you walk, or how frequently. Do you feel better after a Zumba class, a weight training class, or aqua aerobics? Maybe belly dancing or biking are more your speed. If you're suffering from severe fatigue and exhaustion, move your body gently with realistic goals so as not to worsen your fatigue, but see how it feels to get your blood flowing a little. Exercise doesn't necessarily mean being in constant motion; it can be as gentle as taking a walk, gardening, or splashing around in a pool.

Many find that being in an exercise class makes a difference, as the socialization is an added boost to positivity and good health. Find something that works for you and then just make it a point to show up. Don't think about it, don't allow yourself to make excuses, just show up and let the instructor take it from there. Committing to a walking or running schedule with a friend is another great way to stay motivated and socialize at the same time. Motivation is hard in the beginning, so I want to introduce you to this interesting research on how to get and stay motivated to exercise.

Finding the Motivation to Exercise

The problem with motivation is that we often make exercise a "should" instead of a "want." For many people, exercising for health is not a good enough reason to get out of the office chair, or off the sofa. With most of the population struggling with overstuffed schedules, people will only fit in what they feel is absolutely necessary.

Research psychologists say we need an emotional hook to compel us to stay physically active. **The solution is not to exercise for health reasons, but because it makes your life better *now*.** Find what's enjoyable about exercising for you, and use that as your incentive to keep going. For instance, a busy working mom can use a walk with her kids as a way to exercise and spend time with her children, while a busy stay-at-home mom can use a walk to get some time away from her kids – having to walk a dog is also a good motivator.

I know a woman who takes long walks to fulfill a life-long dream of taking photos during her walks to use as inspiration for paintings she will create later. Another woman uses morning walks to socialize with a friend. Exercising in the morning can boost your energy and mood for the rest of the day. If you're unhappy with your weight, you'll find that regular exercise makes you more appreciative of your body.

There are a number of emotional benefits to help motivate you to integrate exercise into your life. Here are some significant reasons to get moving:

- Sleep better at night
- Feel less depressed
- Overcome anxiety
- Relieve stress
- Boost energy and productivity
- Cope more effectively with frustrations
- Enjoy the natural high from physical exertion
- Enhance self-esteem

Perhaps most important of all, find ways to turn your exercise into play-time; scientists have found that other species of intelligent animals, such as dolphins, chimps, and otters, play throughout their adult lives as a way to stay active and socially connected. Unfortunately, many Americans work long hours and have lost touch with the importance of play in their lives, including the stress relief it can bring.

A life of all work and no play (or all television and no play) makes us vulnerable to stress-related diseases, depression, interpersonal violence, and addiction, according to Stuart Brown, MD, author of **Play: How it Shapes the Brain, Opens the Imagination and Invigorates the Soul**, and founder of The National Institute of Play.

Have you forgotten how to play? Recall how you played as a child, and how good it felt. Now consider the numerous options you have available to you, and then experiment with the playful activities that appeal to you or sound like fun. Your joyful bliss could be roller-skating, yoga, horseback riding, shooting baskets, swimming, or playing fetch with Rover. The objective is to forget you're engaging in a powerful form of stress relief because you're having so much fun.

The Elements of Successful Play

Successful play is more a state of mind than a specific activity, and the health benefits go well beyond stress relief. Regular play will make you feel better about yourself, stimulate brain activity, enable you to transform negative experiences, boost creativity and imagination, and help you connect with others.

Do you remember when you were a child with no limitations or inhibitions? Every day was an opportunity to experience something new, an opportunity to learn about something that was not previously part of your world. You would innocently open yourself to this experience in a welcoming way. What happened, as you got older? It's not uncommon to reduce the amount of time we spend playing as we grow older, thankfully it's relatively easy to regain the benefits of making sure we make time in our lives to play.

Regular play makes people happier, and happiness is a great antidote to stress. It's so important to make time to play, have fun, relax, refocus, and have a good time.

Real play has the following qualities:

- All consuming and fun.
- Relaxing, and at the same time stimulating for the body and mind.
- It takes place separate from the rest of your life (a basketball court, the roller rink, a favorite trail, or your back yard).
- Play is about exuberance and releasing negative feelings.
- It requires freedom—you do it because it is enjoyable.
- Play is enjoyed for its own sake.

It may be more important now than ever before to give yourself permission to play. I know, I know, you can barely get through dinner, let alone find time to play. But as you do this program and become more vibrant and glowing, incorporating play into your life will start to seem more natural and possible.

You were created for abundant joy! Your mojo is starting to come back. YOU GO, GIRLFRIEND!

Play, defined.
"To engage in activity for enjoyment and recreation rather
than a serious or practical purpose."
Synonyms: amuse oneself, have fun, enjoy

- Develop a strong sense of faith. Consistently participate in a spiritual, religious, or philosophical practice.

- Practice optimism. Increase your positivity and possibilities thinking. Adopting a few small strategies can add up to significant gains in your motivation and sense of well-being.

- Be grateful. Think of something that makes you feel better—a sunny beach, victorious moment, or good memory—upon waking each morning and when experiencing a setback. Remember times in your life when you were healthy and happy. Embrace all that is going well in your life right now.

- Maintain social connections. Develop and nurture positive friendships. In those with life-threatening illnesses, this has been shown to improve the odds of survival by 50 percent. Join a group in order to meet other people struggling with the same health challenges.

- Be active. Get physical. Although CrossFit or Zumba may not be possible for someone struggling with a chronic illness, research shows physical activity relieves stress, enhances a positive outlook and helps with healing.

- Play regularly. Get in touch with the childlike part of yourself and find activities that you find relaxing and fun.

CHAPTER 10

BUILDING PIECE-MEAL:
Eat Well For Optimal Health

 Suffering forces us to change. We don't like change, and most of the time we fear it and fight it. We would like to remain in emotionally familiar places, even though sometimes those places are not healthy for us. On occasion, the suffering is so great that we have to give up. We surrender the old and begin anew. Often it is a pain we experience that leads us not only to a different life but a richer and more rewarding one."

Dennis Wholey

By the time we hit our 40s, most women feel bludgeoned to death by complicated and conflicting dietary advice. I can look back on my life and mark the passage of time based on what size I wore, and what diet I was on—Weight Watchers, the Ornish diet, the HCG diet, juice fasting, Jenny Craig, etc. Sound familiar? It is a sad and demeaning reflection for an otherwise smart, motivated, and accomplished individual like myself. But I know I'm not alone; look at Oprah and the millions of American women who define themselves based on their weight. You know what I mean: "I ate a dessert so I'm 'bad'. I stuck to my diet so I'm 'good'." How many of your days have been ruined by the number on the bathroom scale?

The fact that it gets harder for most women to lose weight after 40 doesn't help matters. Hormonal fluctuations, chronic stress, and a lifetime of yo-yo dieting can be enough to tip your body into a full-out rebellion, refusing to budge, quite literally, an inch. This is not the time to punish or loathe your body, but rather to listen to it. Your body's ability to deal with excess fat says a great deal about your overall health. You can starve your body into submission in your 20s, but not so much after 40, without getting poor results or repercussions. **This is the time to nurture the beloved temple that is your body, so that it will gracefully carry you through the next part of your life.**

This chapter is about nutrition, it's about food choices and what you eat, it's not specifically about weight loss, we've already addressed that – although losing pounds will often be a happy "side-effect." You already know how to diet; this is about *eating for optimum health,* eating to stabilize the systems in your body, and to calm inflammation and hormonal chaos. Only when you understand how to heal your body with food will you have the tools needed for genuine fat release, if this is appropriate for you. Come with me ThyroSisters, to learn the rules for eating in ways that will nourish, support, and help heal your body.

First Things First: Out With the Junk

So here's the part where I tell you to ditch the junk food. Maybe you already have, if so, bravo! Or maybe you haven't, but you've been told to a million times. Here's the part where you decide whether you want to live out the rest of your life as a strong, healthy, mentally capable person, or as an unhealthy, slowly decaying, and degenerating one. No, I really am not exaggerating.

If you are still eating most of your meals out (or out of a box), if you think a muffin and Grande Mocha Carmel Peppermint Frappuccino qualifies for breakfast, or of you slug down a Diet Coke or energy drink, then this section is particularly important for you. Many women need more information about how to shop for and prepare healthy meals. In this section you are going to learn how to think about and approach eating from a new, different, and exciting perspective.

So what do I mean by *whole foods*? Whole foods describe food in its natural state, food that isn't refined or processed and is free of added ingredients, such as salt or sugar. I'll be honest, when you first start eating whole foods there may be a part of your brain that screams for the titillation that comes from ingesting lab-made flavors, colors, and textures designed to trigger an addiction to them. Research shows that rats react to junk food like human heroin addicts (Sanders, 2009).There's a carefully engineered reason why one Oreo or one Dorito is never enough. But by supplying your body with the right foods in the right amounts (including eating sufficient healthy fats), you can naturally eliminate the cravings for unhealthy foods.

A Whole Food Eating Plan

Many people honestly have no idea what eating a whole foods diet really means. That's okay, American culture is not exactly built around eating one. Some of us were the original latchkey kids, left to fend for ourselves with a pantry full of Ho-Ho's and Twinkies while our moms were at work. We also saw the introduction of the microwave, the snack food industry, and the explosion of fast-food restaurants. We Boomers, and those who came after us, are the true products of years of industrialized eating. Over our lifetime, obesity has grown to affect 30 percent of the population (Hurt RT, 2012). The percentage of people ages 45-54 diagnosed with diabetes has increased 118 percent since 1980 (Centers for Disease Control and Prevention, 2013). And circulatory diseases affect more than 83,000 Baby Boomers, up from 23,760 in the previous generation (U.S. Department of Health and Human Services, 2014).

But it doesn't have to be that way. It's not too late to turn your health around or even to prevent poor health altogether. Here's an introduction to a different approach, embracing and eating whole foods that will satisfy, heal and keep your body healthy.

Proteins

As much as possible choose meats and other animal products from animals raised the way nature intended, outdoors in the sunshine. Pasture-raised meats are not only easier on the planet; they have a much better nutrient profile. Your best sources are from farmer's markets and food co-ops, or through food buying clubs (see appendix for resources). To save money, it's worth investing in a freezer and buying meat in bulk directly from the farmer. If locally raised grass-fed meats are not available, do the best you can within your budget. Here are guidelines in choosing healthy protein sources:

Meat

- **Beef:** Beef from cattle that are grass-fed and not grain-finished, has the optimal balance of essential fatty acids, in addition to conjugated linoleic acids, anti-oxidants, vitamin D, and other important nutrients. Cattle are not designed to eat grain; although it fattens them up it also harms their health and the quality of the meat. If you cannot obtain grass-fed beef, another good resource is organic beef, which is free of hormones and antibiotics. Conventionally raised beef is a last choice.
- **Pork:** As with beef, look for pork raised by local farmers, without hormones and antibiotics. Ideally the pigs will have been allowed outdoors to graze.
- **Lamb:** Look for lamb raised on a pasture.
- **Poultry:** Chickens, turkey, and ducks produce the healthiest meat and eggs when they are allowed outdoors to eat insects and grasses. This is called "pastured poultry," and you can also find "pastured eggs" from local farmers. Chickens allowed to eat grass will produce eggs much higher in omega-3 essential fatty acids, and other nutrients. Organic, free-range poultry is the next best option.
- **Fish:** Wild, deep-water fish is your best option. Farmed fish are fed low quality feed that often has added coloring, a higher contamination of pollutants, and an increased risk of disease. Wild fish is also higher in omega-3s, and other nutrients.

Other Protein Sources

- **Nuts:** The ideal option is organic raw nuts. Many people like to soak or sprout their nuts to make them more digestible and nutrient-rich. To do this, pour nuts into a large bowl, add a liberal amount of salt and cover completely with water. For more information read, Nourishing Traditions by Sally Fallon.

- **Dairy:** Not everyone can eat dairy products as it may trigger an immune response, something you can determine through an elimination-provocation diet or lab testing. However, if you do tolerate dairy products, choose organic dairy from pastured cows, goats, or sheep. At the very least, look for dairy that is free of the rBST hormone, which increases the risk of breast cancer.

- **Soy:** Many vegetarians use soy as their main protein source, but newer research shows that this government-subsidized, genetically modified, and heavily sprayed legume can be problematic. Soy is a powerful goitrogen, meaning it inhibits thyroid function, which can slow down metabolism and hinder fat burning. Soy is also very allergenic for many people. Its abundance of phytoestrogens makes it attractive to women with symptoms of low estrogen (although the other risks still apply), but soy can spell disaster for other hormonal imbalances.

Soy Choices That ARE Good for You!

The process of fermenting soy into gluten free soy sauce, miso, tempeh, or natto neutralizes many of the harmful properties, making these foods safe to eat in moderation.

Fats

Fats have recently gone through a public relations makeover. After having been dragged through the mud for the last few decades and blamed for numerous health problems, it turns out they were taking the rap for the true villains – sugars and high-carbohydrate foods.

Your body needs fat. Your hormones are made of fat. Your brain is made of fat. Fat is what kills cravings for sugar. In my experience, a low-fat diet is a super highway to a mega-binge…or two, or three, or shoot; I just gained back all the weight I lost on that *bleepity-bleep* low-fat diet!

In cooking food, use only healthy, natural fats such as olive oil, butter, or ghee (clarified butter for the dairy intolerant), heavy cream, coconut oil, avocado oil, salmon, or duck fat. Fat is wonderful as a 'slow-burning log' for the body, keeping blood sugar stable and metabolism boosted. If done the right way, eating healthy fats can help your body burn excess fat.

Humans evolved consuming animal fats and when eaten as part of a balanced whole foods diet, they work well to support hormonal balance. Worried about developing heart disease? Then avoid sugars and carbohydrates, which are highly inflammatory and damaging to the arterial walls.

By avoiding vegetable oils and eating healthy fats, you will take in more essential omega-3 fatty acids and reduce your consumption of omega-6 fats, which cause inflammation. The best sources of omega-3 fatty acids include fatty fish (such as salmon and tuna), cod liver oil, egg yolks from properly fed hens, and organ meats from grass-fed animals.

Not all "Natural" Fats are Good for You!

In fact, some are downright dastardly. Avoid the highly unstable polyunsaturated oils made from canola, safflower, sunflower, corn, or soybeans. Once processed these oils become toxic free radicals that disrupt metabolism and cause inflammation in the body.

Also avoid hydrogenated and partially hydrogenated oils, which wreak havoc on many bodily functions and are linked to obesity, diabetes, and dementia. Don't let your kids eat them either, because they become part of the brain and negatively affect its ability to function.

Hormone Health Depends on Good Fats

Healthy hormone production depends on essential fatty acids (EFAs). You have probably heard about fish oil, krill oil, flaxseed oil, evening primrose oil, and black currant seed oil. EFAs are also abundant in cold-water fish and in many raw, unprocessed nuts and seeds. EFAs not only contribute nutrients for healthy hormones but are also needed for good brain function and communication between cells.

Your brain is nearly 60% fat, so you need to feed it fat. Fatty acids are among the most crucial molecules that determine the brain's integrity and ability to perform. Your brain also depends on the protective layer around your neurons, the omega-3 neuronal membrane, where numerous proteins and complex molecules required for transmitting and receiving nerve signals are located (Chang CY, 2009). EFAs, particularly omega-3 fatty acids, are important for brain development and have been shown to possess antidepressant and neuroprotective properties (Robinson JG, 2010). Some EFAs, like dietary decosahexaenoic acid (DHA), have specific jobs, such as ensuring optimum function of the retina and visual cortex. In the average American diet EFA deficiencies are estimated to affect up to 90 percent of the population (Fit Day, 2000-2013). This is mostly due to the consumption of junk food loaded with vegetable oil.

It's important to take a well-rounded fish oil based, high-potency, high-quality EFA supplement to support your hormone and brain health. If you have insulin resistance, your body cannot properly metabolize the EFAs in flax, evening primrose, or black currant seed oil, which is why fish oil is recommended. How do you know if you are taking high-quality essential fatty acids? If you put one of your fish oil capsules in the freezer and it freezes, it is not good. Oil should not freeze. Also, most people do not take enough fish oil. The average EFA capsule contains only 1,000 mg, so most people should take at least 5 to 6 capsules of fish oil daily.

Eating a sufficient amount of healthy fats is also instrumental in stabilizing blood sugar, which is key to balancing hormones. Fats also curb cravings for sugar. As long as you are not loading up on carbohydrates, eating fats will not make you fat – unless you overeat. It is the consumption of excess carbohydrates, which convert into triglycerides for fat storage that make us fat and throws our hormones out of whack.

When buying and consuming fats, the most healthful options are:
- Olive oil

- Coconut oil
- Butter
- Palm oil
- Ghee (clarified butter)
- Duck fat
- Bacon fat
- Other animal fats

The saturated fats (animal fats, coconut oil and palm oil) are stable at high temperatures, and can be safely used for cooking and frying. If the oil you're using starts to smoke you have cooked it at too high a temperature, making it unstable and unhealthy. Toss it out and start over.

Trans Fats Shrink Your Brain

About 60 percent of the brain is made up of fat, which comes from fats consumed in the diet. **Research shows that a diet high in trans fats shrinks the brain and increases the risk of dementia** (Carolinas Thyroid Institute). Trans fats are found in fast foods, processed foods, margarine, shortening, chips, flaky pastries, lots of fried foods, and many popular convenience foods. They can be identified on a list of ingredients as *hydrogenated or partially hydrogenated oil.*

When trans fats become part of the cells and nerve sheaths, they replace vital brain fats, such as DHA, an essential omega-3 fatty acid. As a result, cellular communication suffers, the cells degenerate, brain volume shrinks, memory and cognition suffer, and hormone function suffers. Research shows that trans fats also contribute to clogging the veins and arteries; which inhibits blood flow to the brain and robs it of oxygen and vital nutrients, another factor that shrinks the brain and negatively affects its overall function.

But there's good news ThyroSisters! Study participants who ate foods high in vitamins B, C, D, E and omega-3 fatty acids were found to have larger, healthier brains than their junk-food eating peers (Carolinas Thyroid Institute). These are nutrients easily found in all vegetables, fruits, fish, and raw nuts and seeds. **Eating a whole foods diet protects the brain from shrinkage and decline.** The study subjects who ate a diet abundant in these nutrients consistently scored better on mental performance tests and showed less decline in overall brain function. A diet that includes leafy green vegetables, seafood, eggs, olive oil, avocado, colorful fruits and veggies, nuts, and grass-fed or organic meat provides essential building materials for your brain and cell membranes.

Reasons to Develop a "Veggie Habit"

If there is one thing most Americans are guilty of, it's not eating enough veggies or fresh fruit. It's true that eating fresh produce sometimes requires more work than grabbing a bagel or zapping a pizza pocket. (Of course, apples are a ready-to-go snack!) In many cases produce has to be washed, chopped, seasoned, and cooked in some kind of appetizing way. But developing a good vegetable habit is like developing any other good habit. It takes patience, planning, and discipline in the beginning, but then it makes you feel so good you can't imagine living without it.

For the hormonally challenged, developing a healthy, consistent vegetable habit is of utmost importance in preventing cancer. Plentiful fiber in the diet helps clear the body of excess estrogens that can metabolize into a more toxic form; thus increasing the risk of getting breast or uterine cancer. Excess estrogen leaves the body through the bowel; eating plenty of vegetable fiber means healthy bowel movements for most people. (If your bowels become impacted by fiber, I suggest seeing a doctor.)

If you suffer from constipation, this also allows more time for the toxic form of estrogen to be re-absorbed and sent back into circulation in your body, which increases the chances of stimulating breast tissue to develop cancer. Both constipation and poor bowel function also promote the overgrowth of harmful bacteria in the gut, which can take estrogen that is bound for excretion and send it back into the bloodstream.

Lack of fiber also congests the liver, our main detoxifying organ. The liver helps maintain hormonal balance by ridding the body of excess hormones, and metabolizing the toxic forms that are harmful.

Take advantage of all the healthful benefits of fiber by filling your plate with good quality, nutrient-dense vegetables at every meal. Yes, even breakfast. If you tolerate eggs well, a veggie scramble tastes great. Try cooking up breakfast sausage with a side of veggies. Soup made from healthy ingredients is a lovely way to start the day in winter.

The benefits of developing a good veggie habit go far beyond providing optimal nutrition to our bodies. The extra chewing required forces us to eat more slowly, which studies have shown aids in both digestion and weight loss. Shopping for local, organic produce also helps tune us into the changing seasons, and keeps our diets varied and interesting. Eating plenty of produce also helps you stay hydrated, due to the high water content of vegetables.

What About Green Drinks?

Many green drinks or supplements advertise themselves as a substitute for eating vegetables. Don't be lulled into this claim. Although a good quality green drink has its benefits, and IS better than no veggies, nothing replaces the real thing.

Here are a few tips for making good fruit and veggie choices.

- **Vegetables:** Choose organic vegetables that are fresh and bright in color, such as dark green lettuces, broccoli, carrots, and green beans. Avoid potatoes and corn (technically corn is a grain) since they will send your blood sugar on a roller coaster ride.
- **Fruits:** Eating too much fruit can be a problem if you're prone to blood sugar swings. Avoid fruit juices, which contain too much sugar. Aim for moderate amounts of low-sugar fruits, such as berries, grapefruit, young coconut, or avocado.
- The organic produce section, or your local farmer's market, has a variety of colorful fruits and vegetables to choose from.
- Experiment with new recipes and a variety of seasonings, and different vegetable combinations. Well-prepared veggies are enormously satisfying; they taste good, are inexpensive, and you enjoy the satisfaction of eating food that keeps your body happy and healthy.

- Don't overlook the benefits of cauliflower. This amazingly versatile vegetable has a neutral taste and can be prepared in many delicious ways.

Considerations for Healthy Eating

The USDA Food Pyramid tells us to eat a diet that includes large amounts of grains. I can tell you that if you eat like the pyramid suggests, you will end up looking like one!

The food pyramid was designed primarily to sell tax-payer-subsidized grains back to the American public, not to promote our good health. Also these grains have been bred, genetically modified, and processed to the point that they bear little resemblance to what our ancestors ate. Grains are primarily what farmers feed to fatten up their livestock before slaughter, and they have the same effect in humans.

The Advantages of Healthy Salt

Conventional table salt and the salt used in processed foods, is a refined product processed at high temperatures, which removes vital minerals that are replaced with additives, anti-caking agents, and even sugar. We have been told for years to avoid salt, but in truth the moderate use of the right kind of salt is a key component of a healthy diet.

High quality salt, such as sea salt or pink Himalayan salt, contains more than 100 balanced minerals. However, if you have high blood pressure, you should minimize the amount of salt in your diet while you work on lowering your blood pressure. If you have low blood pressure, salt may help move it up to more normal levels. (Normal blood pressure is 120/80; deviations of more than 10 points are problematic. High blood pressure raises your risk for stroke, and low blood pressure doesn't deliver enough blood into your brain and tissues.)

Why Water is So Important

One of the hardest things to get used to as a health practitioner is how some people just never drink water. Instead, they live on coffee, energy drinks, or sodas, and some have told me they don't even like drinking water. That's like not enjoying breathing air!

Water is vital to every cell, organ, gland, and system in your body. Dehydration can impair detoxification and elimination, and make your blood sticky, which 'gums up' the cardiovascular system. Unfortunately, water contamination can be a problem; tap water often contains pathogens and significant levels of poisonous compounds, such as lead, copper, and other metals. To be safe, tap water should be filtered to remove heavy metals and impurities. Well water should be tested and filtered if necessary.

The problem with filtering is that it also removes the good minerals, so you may need to replenish electrolytes in the water you drink. Also, if you find that water goes right through you, this is an indication that you may have an electrolyte imbalance. (Note that other factors can cause frequent urination.)

A Recipe to Replenish Electrolytes

Add ¼ teaspoon of sea salt to one quart of water. You may want to add a little bit of lemon juice and a few drops of stevia (a natural sweetener) to improve the taste.

You can also add ¼ teaspoon of a commercial liquid trace mineral solution. If you add an electrolyte mix to your water, make sure it does not contain sugar or an artificial sweetener.

Keep Your Blood Sugar Balanced

It's difficult to drive down the road, watch TV, flip through a magazine, or walk through a mall without constantly being tantalized with something sweet to eat. We've got holidays that revolve around sugary treats, and days filled with consuming bottomless sodas, sugary breakfast cereals, pastries, and desserts. Americans consume, on average, more than 150 pounds of sweetener each year! (NH DHHS-DPHS)

The rise of chronic diseases around the world can be traced to the growing consumption of sugar and processed foods. Sugar is an addictive drug and many are hooked on the high it delivers. In addition, sugar is highly profitable for food corporations. My view is that we have strayed too far from our ancestral diets, when sweets were an occasional delicacy, and we now pay the price with our health.

Why is Sugar Such a Problem?

For women, **the problems of eating too much sugar often show up during perimenopause and menopause in the form of impaired hormone function.** How much sugar or carbohydrates you eat profoundly affects your hormones and, therefore, your transition into menopause. You may be able to glide through your youth seemingly unscathed by an addiction to carbs or sugar, but perimenopause is often when the "chickens come home to roost."

Perhaps your previous hormonal imbalances were minor or mundane—PMS, irregular periods, sore boobs, or acne. Then suddenly you're trying to cope with insomnia, fatigue, depression, anxiety, thinning hair, memory loss, bone loss, or high blood pressure, all symptoms of a significant hormonal imbalance, partly due to poor food choices.

Mother Nature created our bodies to live off the land and survive famines, not to feast on sweets. In fact, only one percent of our pancreas is dedicated to responding to excess sugar levels. *Did you know that the human body requires only about a teaspoon of sugar in the bloodstream at any one time?* This is a level we easily meet by consuming vegetables daily. When we overindulge in eating carbohydrates, whether it's dessert, pasta, potatoes, or rice, our pancreas must secrete a large dose of insulin to control the elevated blood sugar levels that are the result.

Over time the constant onslaught of too much sugar and too many carbs overwhelms the pancreas, which then secretes increasing amounts of insulin, sending your blood sugar into a nosedive. This is when you feel jittery, light-headed, irritable, or spaced out. Refueling with more sugar makes you feel amazing (for a short time) and then sends your blood sugar levels skyrocketing, repeating the cycle yet again, and yanking your body's systems back and forth like a dog shaking a toy animal.

After a while the body's cells, bludgeoned by constant insulin surges, 'lock the doors' and become insulin resistant. At this point the cells do not allow insulin, and the glucose they're carrying, to enter. As a result glucose levels in the bloodstream remain high, damaging arterial walls and the brain. When glucose can't get into the cells, the resulting high blood sugar leads to water retention, fatigue, and weight gain.

When glucose remains in the bloodstream it turns into triglycerides, which the body stores as fat. Turning glucose into triglycerides demands a lot of energy, which will cause you to feel tired after eating. This partly explains why a big holiday meal, a giant plate of pasta, or a big bowl of ice cream puts some people into a mini-coma. I like Dr. Kharrazian's rule of thumb: If you feel sleepy or crave sugar after eating, you just ate too many carbohydrates.

How to Control Blood Sugar Issues

It is often impossible to manage a blood sugar disorder unless you eat a healthy breakfast that includes high-quality protein. Your body requires protein in the morning to break the night long fast and support healthy blood sugar levels. Chose eggs, nuts, breakfast meats such as turkey or chicken sausage, or even some of last night's dinner. ThyroSisters, if you skip breakfast you depend on stress hormones to fuel you, which puts healthy hormone function on the back burner.

Even if you feel nauseous upon waking—a common side effect of a blood sugar disorder—eating a healthy, protein based breakfast is critical. And eating a high protein breakfast is likely to relieve your nausea. Force yourself to do it; you'll most likely get positive results. If you have hypoglycemia, you should never miss meals, as it will make your symptoms even worse.

Gaining control over your blood sugar issues has some unexpected positive benefits, to include increased happiness! I have seen many women combat chronic depression by balancing blood sugar and getting regular exercise. This is because blood sugar highs and lows cause an imbalance in serotonin, which is our brain's 'feel-good' chemical.

Another benefit of balanced blood sugar is improved memory. The links between blood sugar imbalances and dementia are so well established that some scientists call Alzheimer's disease "Type 3 diabetes" (de le Monte SM, 2008). Insulin resistance and insulin surges are very damaging to the brain. Eating a diet designed to keep blood sugar stable and getting regular exercise significantly reduces your risk of developing memory loss, dementia, or Alzheimer's disease.

Chase Away the Sugar Blues

So how do you get a grip on a tenacious sugar addiction? First, make sure to consume enough vegetable fiber, protein, and healthy fats (such as coconut oil) and that you are digesting these fats. How do you know if you are digesting fats correctly? Well…this is a smelly answer! You may experience flatulence yes, my sweet friend, and also bloating after eating unhealthy or undigested fats. You may notice stool changes, such as diarrhea, because of undigested fats, or foul smelling stools that float. Stools may appear very pale because bile salts are responsible for the brown color of normal stools, and when there are undigested fats the stool color is lighter. Aren't you glad you asked?

Keep your energy levels stable and you will be less likely to eat impulsively. Feeling hungry can be a dark enemy on this quest for health, which is why I hate low-calorie and low-fat diets. There is no bigger set up for a food binge, or eating something unhealthy or high in calories, than hunger. Binging while on a low-fat diet is not poor will power, laziness, or a shameful act. It is the very natural and normal response of a hungry brain.

The best way to avoid hunger is to eat the right kinds of foods and to eat often enough that your brain is never starved for energy. Next time you have a craving, or feel like you're going to cheat, don't reach for sugar or carbs; eat a little protein instead, like a handful of nuts or a hardboiled egg. Eating carbs will trigger cravings for more. Many people experience a substantial decrease in their cravings by giving up sugary and starchy foods.

I see patients get the best results with the Paleo diet. *Primal Blueprint* and the *Paleo Solution* are both very informative books about this way of eating. Both diets encourage eating more like our ancestors did, which didn't include frozen, genetically modified, or processed foods. The basic premise is to eat primarily vegetables, meat, seafood, nuts, and seeds. I urge you to read about Paleo diets to learn more. But be wary of dogma, listen to your body, and have lab tests done regularly to check that you're getting the results you're looking for.

One question that often comes up is, "How many carbs *should* I eat?" There is controversy over this subject in the Paleo world. It's easy to get healthy carbs from sweet potatoes, fruits, nuts, and the occasional serving of whole grains or legumes. If you feel sleepy or crave carbs after eating a meal with no carbs, you may have insulin resistance, in which case you will benefit from supplements and exercise.

Some people find they can gauge how many carbs to eat based on whether they're losing weight, sleeping well, and managing inflammation. Pay close attention to your body, it is speaking to you all the time. Food is either your medicine or it's your poison; it's your choice.

Want to Learn More About Your Daily Carb Intake? Try This!

Many people find that eating no more than 50 grams of "net" carbohydrates a day produces amazing results: increased energy, resolved health complaints, happy hormones, and weight loss. Net carbohydrates are the grams of carbs, excluding the fiber.

Record what you eat each day on a smart phone app such as www.myfitnesspal.com (Ignore the app's default goal settings, which are designed for USDA Pyramid-eaters). Tracking your intake of carbs and fiber may lead to some surprises. You may find you've been eating 50 grams in just one snack or dessert. One can of soda, for example, contains 40 grams of carbs! One cup of plain pasta contains almost 80 grams of carbs. A better choice would be an apple (7 grams, net), a half cup of sweet potato (14 grams), or 1 cup of broccoli (6 grams).

You may need more net carbs in certain situations, for instance if you play sports or exercise often. On the other hand, you may need fewer if you have stubborn weight loss resistance.

Secrets Whispered to a ThyroSister

If eating fat makes you feel nauseous, gives you diarrhea, or makes you burp, you most likely suffer from a congested gallbladder and are not digesting fats properly. In this case you need some gallbladder support to include dandelion root, milk thistle seed extract, ginger root, phosphatidylcholine, or lipase. If your gallbladder has been removed, I also recommend taking ox bile with meals that contain fat, in order to maintain good gut health.

* Learn all you can about how to eat well! Get together with other like-minded ThyroSisters for healthy ideas, information and support. Join us online at www.ThyroSisters.com

* Look for good quality fish markets in your area, or visit www.vitalchoice.com

* A good source of high-quality, organic meat is: www.uswellnessmeats.com

* Visit Cyrex Labs www.cyrexlabs.com to learn about blood test panels that identify gluten-associated, cross-reactive foods, and other food sensitivities.

* If digesting meat is difficult for you, you may be deficient in hydrochloric acid (HCl), a stomach acid necessary to digest protein. If you are deficient in HCl, supplemental HCl can be profoundly therapeutic. (Do not use HCl if you have an ulcer.)

* Prep vegetables ahead of time and store in the fridge, but not for too long. This way they are ready to go for a quick salad or stir-fry.

CHAPTER 11
BUILDING YOUR ENVIRONMENT:
Reducing Exposure to External Toxins

> **" Be careful the environment you choose for it will shape you. "**
>
> *W. Clement Stone*

I'd like you to do an exercise. After reading this sentence, I'd like you to close your eyes and imagine all of the electronic devices you come into contact with in any given day: the microwave in the kitchen, your computer and cell phone, television and stereo. Go ahead and close those beautiful eyes of yours. How many electronic devices do you count in your everyday environment?

This is an issue seriously undermining our health that didn't even exist 20 or 30 years ago. I'm talking about environmental toxins and "electrosmog" pollution from artificially generated frequency waves, coming from your cell phone, big screen TV, and tablets. Just what exactly is this electrosmog? Our electrical devices are not completely efficient with their use of energy; almost every device gives off some sort of unused energy. It's like runoff water that goes into the storm drain when you water your lawn too much, only electrosmog accumulates in the air all around us. Eventually, it may end up in our bodies.

Electrical appliances radiate three types of energy: electrical impulses, electromagnetic waves, and scalar waves. Electrical impulses power devices to include mobile phones, toothbrushes and TVs. Electromagnetic waves are sort of a wild energy used in microwave ovens that can destroy the nutritional value of foods. They are also responsible for that warm sensation on your ear from the cell phone. Scalar waves cannot be destroyed nor created, only blocked or super imposed on each other. The good news is that they can be focused, ordered and harmonized as they carry basic information which make ordered life possible. The cells of the human body communicate through scalar waves, sending out signals to other cells, sort of like truckers with CB radios.

Typical symptoms of electrosmog exposure are chronic fatigue, weak knees, back pain, the inability to think clearly, memory lapses, cold feet and diffuse chronic pain in the lower abdomen. The biggest "aha" is being sent to the psychiatrist because of your "psychosomatic" illness!

Now, close your eyes again and imagine you are standing in your bathroom. Look around at the bathing products in the shower, the beauty products in the cabinet, and the cleaning products under the sink. Most of these products are filled with chemicals and man-made materials that are in some way toxic or inflammatory to our bodies. Today we live in an environment that includes tens of thousands of man-made synthetic chemicals, only a few of which have been tested for safety.

Toxic chemicals are frequently found in our makeup, hair and body products, household cleaning products, plastics, furniture, flooring, countertops, and paint. It is pretty much impossible to live completely chemical-free today, and many of these chemicals are now being linked to cancers, brain diseases (to include Alzheimer's and Parkinson's), hormonal imbalances, poor liver function, and many more. In addition, many chemicals and plastics in the environment contain xenoestrogens, synthetic chemicals that mimic and compete with estrogen, potentially creating hormonal imbalances with symptoms of estrogen dominance; thus increasing the risk of cancer in breasts and reproductive organs.

Many people regard toxins and electrosmog the way people once regarded germs: as something that doesn't exist because it's not visible to the eye. But **studies continue to validate the health risks and dangers of toxic chemicals and electrosmog.** Increasingly, electrosmog is linked with health risks and complications, to include cancers, brain diseases, sleep problems, and hormonal imbalance.

For the sensitive female body with its complex hormonal structure, the negative health effects of toxins and electrosmog can be overwhelming, especially as hormones begin waning in the middle years, making us even more vulnerable.

Fortunately, there are ways to reduce your sensitivity to environmental chemicals and electro smog. It's not realistic for most of us to escape to a pristine environment free of toxins, cell phone frequencies, and Wi-Fi, but there are ways to help your body become more resistant, which will help buffer it from the damage.

You can learn more about the science and legislation behind electrosmog at www.electrosmogprevention.org/, as well as the American Academy of Environmental Medicine.

Protect Your Body From Chemical Sensitivities

Why are some people chemically sensitive and others aren't? Most people, and many practitioners, mistakenly believe it's because sensitive people have higher levels of toxins in their systems. The fact is that chemically sensitive people are reacting to toxins and heavy metals, while people who are not chemically sensitive do not react.

In today's society we all have fairly high levels of toxins and heavy metals in our systems. Anthropologists have found that even ancient mummies had high levels of heavy metals in their systems, although not the neurotoxins found in dryer sheets or air fresheners! Some people react to toxins or metals in the same ways that people react negatively to gluten, dairy, or pollen. The constant exposure keeps their immune systems in red alert, and soon a cornucopia of unwanted symptoms develop.

The steps needed to reduce sensitivity to toxins in our environment are similar to the ones used to reduce autoimmune flare-ups, previously discussed. One of your best defenses is to keep your glutathione levels boosted. I use an oral liquid liposomal glutathione (a sulfur that is produced in the body that helps enhance all of your antioxidants, to include Vitamin C and E) that is absorbed before it goes through the digestive process.

It's also important to do what you can to avoid as many toxins in your environment as possible. One of the places where you have the most control over allowing chemical toxins to enter your body is in the food you eat. Chose organic, fresh foods instead of processed food as much as possible, and stay away from alcohol. Additionally use lotions, make-up, and soaps that do not contain cancer-causing chemicals such as BHA (butylated hydroxyanisole) and BHT (butylated hydroxytoluene). These are closely related synthetic antioxidants used as preservatives in many lipsticks and moisturizers. DEA (diethanolamine) is used to make cosmetics creamy or sudsy, but is also known to cause liver cancers and precancerous changes in skin and thyroid. Parabens are used widely in cosmetics as a preservative, and are suspected endocrine disrupters that may interfere with male reproductive functions. **The bottom line is this, the fewer toxins you have in your body, the better.**

ThyroSisters, I get it, I know how hard it can be to find natural, low-chemical products, and how expensive. The simple truth is that even if you don't have sensitivity to chemicals, your body still has to work to eliminate them. And your body was meant for so much more! Spending all your body's resources on eliminating toxins is like a gifted cello player working her fingers to the bone washing dishes all day, leaving her too burnt out and tired to share her talent in front of an enthralled audience at night. Wouldn't you rather spend your body's resources on writing the novel you've been thinking about for years, playing with your kids or grandkids, or running a marathon? I know I would!

How to Reduce Your Sensitivity to Chemicals, Electrosmog and Heavy Metals:

- **Defend your body with glutathione.** I recommend a liposomal glutathione liquid that is absorbed through the lining of the stomach. You can also take oral S-acetyl glutathione (a precursor to glutathione), or boost your glutathione levels with N-acetylecysteine, cordyceps, gotu kola, milk thistle extract, L-glutamine, or alpha lipoic acid. Examples of glutathione rich foods are garlic, onions, broccoli, kale, cabbage, walnuts, and lamb. Glutathione helps to eliminate heavy metals and shield the body from environmental toxins.
- **Keep your immune system strong** with D3 and high-quality fish oil supplements, and consistently exercising and getting enough restorative sleep.

- **Dampen inflammation** in the body with curcumin and resveratrol.
- **Pay attention** to what you put into your body. Filter your water and choose organic foods as often as possible.
- Take **liver support** compounds, if needed. If your liver is not working properly, it will backlog poorly metabolized hormones, and other compounds, adding to the toxic burden.
- **EMF & RF Solutions** in Encinitas, California www.emfrf.com, will test your home and property for EMF pollution and suggest remedies. You can also buy a variety of products from www.lessemf.com to protect your home and body.
- **Minimize your exposure** to toxins as much as possible. Ditch the obvious offenders: dryer sheets, air fresheners, scented detergents, scented candles, artificially scented body products, and pesticides.
- **Reduce your exposure** to electrosmog with limited usage of cell phones, tablets, and electrical appliances.

Secrets Whispered to a ThyroSister

Examples of potential environmental triggers include cigarette smoke, pesticides, or benzines in gas fumes. The scents of laundry detergents, perfumes, colognes, aftershave, and fabric softeners are major stimuli for some people. The products we are exposed to regularly that contain toxic chemicals include cleaning products, cosmetics, shampoo, carpeting, tile floors, furniture, clothing, plastics, paint, and nail polish.

It really is impossible not to come in contact with these toxins, and if we are stressed, depleted, imbalanced, or chronically exhausted, our ability to tolerate these chemicals weakens, and we become more susceptible to developing physical damage from them. But there's no need to read this book from under your bed while wearing a hazmat suit! Running labs and adjusting your diet and lifestyle changes are often enough to manage or prevent the effects of these harmful substances.

CHAPTER 12
THE PUZZLE IS SOLVED,
THE REBUILDING IS COMPLETE,
YOUR MOJO IS BACK!

> **"** If we are creating ourselves all the time, then it is never too late to begin creating the bodies we want instead of the ones we mistakenly assume we are stuck with. **"**
>
> *Deepak Chopra*

How to Maintain Your Mojo, Without Going Crazy!

At the beginning of our journey together I introduced Lauren – fatigued, losing her hair, unable to lose weight, constipated, suffering from brain fog, and experiencing painful intercourse due to vaginal atrophy. So perhaps you're wondering what happened to her, was she able to regain her mojo? And if so, how did she do it?

I would love to say that she lived happily ever after with no hiccups, but that would not be keeping it real. Here's how she's really doing… the weight dropped off (23 pounds) her vitality and sense of strength returned, hair stopped falling out, she has a robust bowel movement every day and the relationship with her husband is more intimate than ever!

Yet, she confessed to me that when she started feeling good, she would cheat a little bit here and there, for example eating a little gluten so she wouldn't "hurt her friends' feelings" or skipping taking a few supplements. Sometimes within 72 hours her symptoms would hit hard, often a headache. Other times symptoms would return slowly; the brain fog would start to shadow her thoughts, her weight would start to creep back up (due to inflammation) hot flashes would begin to appear again. Fortunately she knew what to do to regain her previous healthy functioning and get her mojo back once again.

What I so admire about Lauren, and other ThyroSisters that I've been honored to know, is that it is not how many times you go down, it's how many times you get back up! Lauren has learned over time that this Mojo lifestyle is a marathon, not a sprint. For the rest of her life, she'll be managing, monitoring and overseeing her "god-pod", as Kris Carr calls our precious body. You too will learn through this process that you are your own best doctor. There's not to be any beating yourself up, or letting yourself become discouraged, just lean into your faith, get some "me" time without any guilt, chose to be around people you love, exercise, remember to take needed supplements, make sleep a priority, accept yourself exactly as you are.

For many women, giving up favorite foods, going off sugar cold turkey, taking on a new diet, or making exercise a habit is challenging, to say the least! When it comes to making major lifestyle changes, I find that for most people consistent compliance depends on how miserable they've been feeling. **When the pain of the problem outweighs the pain of the solution, change comes more easily.**

When a ThyroSister is fed up with experiencing chronic pain, fatigue, anxiety, insomnia, or depression, fed up with not living life fully – she's far more motivated to exercise, take supplements, give up gluten, or embrace the anti-inflammatory diet, whatever she needs to do to heal. For most of my patients, knowing there are solutions to chronic health problems is exciting news and a huge relief.

Keep in mind that **the journey to good health isn't a straight slope upward, but a gentle trend toward improvement, with peaks and valleys along the way.** Most women will notice progressive signs of improvement, but there will also be backslides, and bad days when you seem to be doing everything right, but still feel lousy. This is often due to your body adjusting to the changes that you're making, to include detoxing your system.

It helps to keep in mind that you are embarking on this journey so you can regain a strong zest for life and the good health to live it fully. I see women get the best results by making changes slowly and carefully "listening" to their body while doing so. It's not uncommon to make changes and then lose sight of the difference that it's making. For example, the negative reaction to eating gluten, after not having had it for a while, can be so severe that the return of symptoms motivates permanent change. Or if you get into an exercise routine and then take time off, feeling antsy, restless, and 'icky' often gets you back on track fast.

On the other hand, sometimes I see patients become completely obsessed with taking on a new, healthy lifestyle, and this has its downside as well. While I applaud enthusiasm, and even offer a little dietary evangelism (nobody can proselytize quite like the happily gluten-free!) I have seen people drive themselves a little insane with efforts to achieve "healthy" eating. Agonizing over every meal, spending hours doing Internet research, obsessing over labels, or worrying too much about each detail of the changes you're making; this isn't going to yield positive results either. Find a reasonable balance that is effective and works for you, and stick with it the best you can.

Embrace and Enjoy Moving Forward

Making your health a priority is rewarding in and of itself. Feeling better physically and mentally, and knowing that you are now the one in charge is a powerfully motivating feeling!

My recommendation is that what's most important is not to obsess about the healthy changes you're making, but to celebrate your progress, pay attention to how you feel, and have lab tests on a regular basis to clinically monitor what's happening in your body.

Throughout this book I have outlined important principles about how to eat well for a healthy immune system, and ways to balance your hormones and brain chemistry. As you continue to make progress and learn more about how your body is responding, you'll discover that the details of what to eat, which supplements work best, and how to stay on track varies from one person to another.

If you stick to the basics that we've discussed in this book, following a whole foods diet, moving your body, and identifying the core cause of your health issues, over time you will figure out what works best for you, and what doesn't. **Remember, good health is all about balance.**

Yes, eating well for your health and happiness can be a tough adjustment in the beginning, but soon it becomes routine and a way of life with results you won't want to give up.

Additional Suggestions for Living a Healthy Lifestyle:
- On weekends, prepare large batches of food to eat during the week.
- Use a grill for quick cooking; just remember not to blacken meat or fish.
- When dining, try to engage with other supportive friends or family members.
- Locate other people who live a healthy lifestyle so that you can do so together.
- Use a slow cooker so a warm meal is waiting for you when you get home from work, and the delicious smells will greet you.
- Chop and store veggies ahead of time, so that sautéing and steaming can be done quickly.
- Find a few spice and herb blends you like in order to quickly season meats, vegetables, and sauces.
- Invest in a good blender (Vita-Mix or Blend Tec) that quickly turn veggies into a smoothie. Just don't add too much fruit.
- Form a cooking co-op with friends, in which you take turns cooking. One person cooks enough for everyone, and you get a night, or several nights off.

The No-Excuses Program

People faced with the prospect of having to make changes can suddenly come up with every excuse in the book for not doing so. This is no way to live; good health means being happy and positive about your choices. It helps to acknowledge your own self-worth, and the fact that you deserve good health. **Do you want to strut your sexy mojo during a lifetime of feeling good?**

My patients who embrace these lifestyle changes do so because they want to feel better, live a long, healthy life, and be who they were created to be. At times they have soldiered on through setbacks and difficulties, but most have grown to love this way of life. Those who accept responsibility for their health see what their new habits have given them—their life. You're worth the effort, that's for sure!

This is a whole new season in your life, and I am so proud of you! I promised in the beginning of this book that I would share with you all that I have learned over the years, and in fact I continue to keep learning. I wrote this book to show you that you can do so much more than survive or suffer through your life; **you can take steps today to live beautifully, inside and out.**

Yes, I'm talking about you. In recapturing and maintaining your mojo, the creative ideas, dreams, and life you know is waiting to burst forth will be able to do so. You were not created for mediocrity; you were created for joy, and to live an innovative, inspirational, exceptional life!

Remember the concepts of "possibility thinking" that we discussed earlier? These ideas are based on the ways you lived life when you were a child; playful, and open to the abundance of life. The good, no the GREAT news is that the result of this healthy lifestyle is freedom! As a result of taking care of your health, you will become increasingly capable and confident. When challenges hit (and they will), you will have the brainpower to think of solutions, the physical strength to hit your knees in prayer, and the emotional clarity to view your life with gratitude.

Make it a point to realize the liberation from anxiety and despair that you will experience because your spirit is alive again, the inner voice that makes you uniquely you; and you will now have the physical fortitude to follow through on your hopes and dreams. Be careful not to view these changes from a place of deprivation, as this will work against you. You are not being deprived or losing out on anything when you are feeling better and thinking more clearly than you have in years! Decide to take a leadership role within yourself, and in doing so you will be an inspiration to others. Go gluten-free with a friend, but don't wait for a friend to start your new life. Rest assured that when you begin to shine, others will follow.

I suggest taking a moment each time before you eat to be grateful for all the people who made it possible to get that luscious plate of healthy food to your table. **The hardest part is now behind you.** You have been empowered with knowledge about why you felt so tired, and reassured that it wasn't all in your head. You now have the knowledge and tools you need to succeed. Now, ThyroSister, it's up to you.

Realistically, you may 'fall off the wagon' every now and then, but I know you have the strength to get back up. It's not how many times you fail ThyroSister; it's how many times you keep getting back up. And baby, they haven't seen anything like you yet!

I wish that I could talk with you over your kitchen table to help you lick your wounds and celebrate your wins. While I can't do that for each and every one of you, there may be another ThyroSister out there who can. That's why I've built an online community just for you at www.ThyroSisters.com. Learn from each other's mistakes. Motivate and encourage each other. Because you are not alone, none of us have to do this on our own.

You will no longer worry that you are crazy, lazy, or finished! ThyroSisters, it's true that what goes on between those pretty ears of yours is so important. Your thoughts and perceptions of your environment, your friends, family, and the challenges are all there to awaken and empower you to lead a truly magical and transformed life.

YOU ARE NOT ALONE!

Keep in mind that you are not alone in healing and reclaiming your mojo. My team of highly trained professionals is available to help you with any aspect of your healing and to answer any questions.

When you contact us, we will roll up our sleeves to show you how to make connections between your symptoms and healing solutions. We will help you with lab testing, supplements, and whatever else you need.

Contact me through my office if I can help or support your journey in any way. Stay tuned to my website where we will keep you updated on the latest health news about hormones, thyroid health, vibrancy, wellness, events, programs, supplements, healing recipes, and more.

Dr. J. Labbe
Email: support@ThyroSisters.com
858-284-9501 Office (PST)

Thank you so much for allowing me to share with you my experiences, knowledge, and stories of women who have gone through what you are going through, and have achieved amazing results. You are not alone, and I wish you major magical mojo in the months and years ahead. Make these the absolute best years of your life!

ACKNOWLEDGEMENTS

I want to thank the following people for their dedication and commitment to helping me complete this book and for supporting my vision to help others live a stronger, more vibrant, mojo-filled life!

Heartfelt thanks to Dr. Juergen Winkler, M. D. for his tireless work. For his passion to treat the whole person's genetic, spiritual, emotional, and physical makeup, instead of just treating the disease. Dr. Neil Neimark, M.D., you have my deepest respect and gratitude. Thank you for your encouragement, wisdom and support.

Ariela Wilcox, thanks for tracking me down and encouraging me by "holding my feet to the fire," and helping me to develop the ThyroSisters vision of commitment to a vibrant life. Elaine Fawcett, thank you for making this project a pleasure to work on and for your insightful ways of communicating the good news that there is a way to have a happy, healthy mid-life. My deepest thanks to Kathryn Rudlin; I had been looking for someone who 'got it,' and me, for years. I am so fortunate and blessed to have your expertise, experience, friendship, and support in this project. Heartfelt thanks to brilliant Jessica, and creative Kat for your extraordinary insight, storytelling, and wisdom. Your support created a profound shift in communication within me that is a treasured gift.

My deepest thanks to my "inside team," directed by Darlene Smith, and Amy Donald, for your amazing drive and commitment to expand our vision for living a healthy life. I am so blessed to work with you. To my thyroid clients who I have learned so much from; I am so honored to have your trust and to be part of your lives. Appreciation to my amazing social media team, especially Penny Sansevieri, for being so wonderfully supportive of my vision and message. To Marcie Smith, Paradigm Design, for her creative eye for design and balance, and razor sharp ability to get the mood across in different mediums. Many thanks to David Davis for his patience, easy personality, and creative genius.

To the American Association of Integrative Medicine profession, I am honored to be a member of such a progressive and informative group. And to my wonderful personal ThyroSisters who have been in the trenches with me. We have laughed, supported each other, cried, dieted, compared beauty tips, lived through births, deaths, marriages, and divorces, and danced our way through the challenges of midlife together.

And finally to mom and dad, who both left this earth too young. The mark you left on people in this world with your unwavering love, dedication and willingness to always care, instruct and love will transcend more than you can imagine. Your influence helped me write some of the principals in this book. Thank you for instilling in me the knowledge that *"I can do all things through Him who gives me strength." (Philippians 4:13)*

ABOUT THE AUTHOR - JONI LABBE, DC, CCN, DCCN

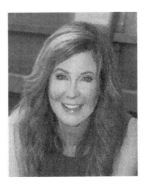

Dr. Labbe is a Board-Certified Clinical Nutritionist and Dr. of Chiropractic, specializing in science-based nutrition, with a specialized focus on hypothyroid, Hashimoto's and women's hormone health. She has successfully helped pre-menopausal and menopausal women regain and maintain their health since 1995. She is a professional speaker, radio personality, fitness expert, and former host of "Healthier Way With Dr. Labbe."

She has earned a Diplomate and Fellow in Nutrition from the American Association of Integrative Medicine and is pursuing a degree in Functional Neurology from the prestigious Carrick Institute. Dr. Labbe is one of the country's leading authorities on thyroid disorders, including Hashimoto's disease. She is the founder of Mojo Thyroid Girlfriends Inc, and creator of the ThyroSisters™ M.V.P. Measurable, Verifiable, Progress, Program. A comprehensive plan for women struggling with hypothyroid, Hashimoto's and hormone imbalances. She has appeared and authored numerous articles and blogs on health, nutrition, and hypothyroid health as seen in Fox Health News, Healthy Times, and KUSI TV.

In her free time, Dr. Labbe enjoys hiking and exploring with her husband in the beautiful surroundings of San Diego. When the opportunity to travel comes, she enjoys learning about other people and cultures, especially as it relates to their indigenous culinary preferences, health and longevity. "Music touches us emotionally, where words alone can't" (Johnny Depp). The power of music, in any form, is one of her passions, especially gospel, jazz, and the blues; favorites are Ray Charles, Billy Holiday, Etta James, and the great Eric Clapton. Laughing with friends and family over a great "tribal meal" is her idea of an evening well-spent. Dr. Labbe provides an excellent example of living vibrantly post-menopause; as in addition she successfully manages her own symptoms of Hashimoto's and Celiac disease. It's her life's mission to help others "lose that voice in your head telling you that you're *crazy, lazy, or finished!*"

CONTACT INFORMATION

ThyroSisters™

Joni Labbe, DC, CCN, DCCN, FCCN

Phone: 858-284-9501

email: support@thyrosisters.com

www.thyrosisters.com

Along with her ThyroSisters MVP Measurable, Verifiable, Progress Program™, Dr. Labbe's approach to health is guided by the principals of rejuvenating and regaining vitality and optimism through identifying and balancing hormones, auto immune, adrenal, thyroid issues, metabolic problems, and brain concerns. Science-based nutritional solutions, detoxifying and cleansing, functional neurology, diet and lifestyle are all addressed in her ThyroSisters™ MVP Program.

About the foreword writer, Dr. Neil F. Neimark:

Dr Neil Neimark, M.D., is a Board-Certified Family Physician, author and speaker who utilizes the foundational principles of functional medicine, along with his focus on the entire person (body, mind and soul) to help patients achieve greater physical health and emotional well-being.

He is the author of the "Mastering Stress" series of books designed to help patients use powerful skills and not just pills to reduce stress, anxiety, worry and depression and reclaim their health, happiness and peace of mind.

Dr. Neil Neimark: www.thebodysoulconnection.com,

www.5minutestressmastery.com, www.theacademyofstressmastery.com

About the preface writer, Dr. Juergen Winkler

Dr. Winkler, MD, is Board Certified in Family Medicine and has maintained an interest in alternative and complementary medicine since medical school. In 1996 he joined the American College for the Advancement in Medicine.

Dr. Winkler has special training in chelating therapy, Insulin Potentiation Therapy (IPT) for cancer treatment, and Mesotherapy for pain management. He is also a member of the American College of Osteopathic Pain Management and Sclerotherapy, Inc. His treatment approach is based on nutrition, heavy metal detoxification, and immune system enhancements. In addition, he treats hormone conditions associated with menopause, hypothyroidism and andropause. Find out more about Dr. Winkler at: www.qfmed.com/

RESOURCES FOR HEALTH

Here are resources for the people, products, and therapies I recommend to ThyroSisters. You can contact my office for more advice and information on supplements, testing, and other resources.

Dr. Joni Labbe, D.C., CCN, DCCN

ThyroSisters MVP Measurable, Verifiable, Progress Program™ www.thyrosisters.com

Dr. Al A. Fallah, DDS, FICCMO

760-730-1600 www.dentistryforsandiego.com/why-choose-fallah.htm

Dr. Richard W. Levak Ph.D

Personality expert, author of books on personality, and former testing psychologist for Survivor, The Amazing Race, Apprentice, Big Brother, and many others. www.drlevak.com

858-755-8717

Institute of Functional Medicine www.functionalmedicine.org

Please refer to their list of doctors around the country to find a practitioner in your area.

Kathryn Rudlin, LCSW

Therapist and author of Ghost Mothers: Healing From the Pain of a Mother Who Wasn't Really There

krudlinlcsw@att.net

www.ghostmothers.com

619-987-5471

Dr. Scott Theirl DC, DACNB, FACFN

Dr. Theirl is a leading board-certified chiropractic neurologist who lectures nationally on topics including brain-based rehabilitation, neurotransmitters, stress physiology, sex hormones, food sensitivities, childhood development delays and insomnia. He is the creator of the Insomnia Insight. www.drtheirl.com 800-385-1655

Dr. Juergen Winkler, M.D.

Physician – Quantum Functional Medicine www.qfmed.com 760-585-4616

Supplements

Apex Energetics: www.apexenergetics.com

Many of the formulas I recommend are created by Dr. Kharrazian for Apex Energetics.

Premiere Research Labs: www.prlabs.com/shop

This company produces excellent nutritional supplements that I use regularly.

NeuroScience: www.neurorelief.com

This company specializes in formulas for brain health. I especially like Kavinace as a natural sleep aid.

ReadiSorb: www.readisorb.com

ReadiSorb makes a liquid liposomal glutathione that is absorbed before it goes through the digestive process. Glutathione is a powerhouse product that is helpful in balancing out auto immune disorders. Go to www.pubmed.gov and search "glutathione" to find over 80,000 articles listed on the key role glutathione plays in healing or stabilizing many diseases.

Numedica: www.numedica.com

Reliable ground breaking formulas of superior quality. They have been recognized for offering the highest quality state of the art supplements.

Biotics: www.bioticsresearch.com

Utilizing "The Best of Science and Nature" to create Superior Nutritional Supplements

Designs for Health: www.designsforhealth.com

Provides comprehensive support through an extensive line of nutritional products.

EnerDMG: www.nutritionalfrontiers.com

DMG by Nutritional Frontiers contains N-Dimethylglycine. By enhancing metabolism, EnerDMG supports the immune, circulatory, cardiovascular, and neurological systems; as well as muscle recovery and endurance. Many of my patients report improved mood and energy while taking it.

NOTE: It's important to work with a health care practitioner who can recommend supplements and formulas based on your individual needs.

Healthy Eating

Cultures for Health: www.culturesforhealth.com
Fermented and cultured foods are an important part of a gut-repair diet. Cultures for Health is an excellent online resource for cultures, recipes, and how-to videos.

US Wellness Meats: www.uswellnessmeats.com
Buying grass-fed meats and products is difficult in some areas of the country. US Wellness Meats offers a wide variety of products that are shipped frozen to your home.

Tropical Traditions: www.tropicaltraditions.com
Tropical Traditions specializes in coconut and other oils, in addition to grass-fed meats and natural products for the home and body.

Animal Welfare Approved: www.animalwelfareapproved.org
Look for AWA labels on meats and other products you buy to ensure that the animal raising process was healthy for the animal. Healthier animals mean healthier animal products.

Local Harvest: www.localharvest.org
Local Harvest helps you find local, seasonal, and community-based produce, no matter where you are in the U.S.

Sustainable Food: www.eatwell.org
Find sustainable food products in your area of the country.

Organic Gardening: www.organicgardening.com
Learn how to grow your own produce organically, or learn tips and tricks for finding organic growers in your area.

Organic Store Locator: www.organicstorelocator.com
Find organic stores anywhere in the United States.

Recommended Reading

Crazy Sexy, Diet. Crazy Sexy Kitchen and Crazy Sexy Cancer Tips: Eat Your Veggies, Ignite Your Spark and Live Like you Mean It by Kris Carr

Kris Carr is a wellness activist and cancer survivor; her book is an excellent source of information and motivation about healthy eating and juicing. You will love her style and tips. She really packs a wallop in her health message, one of my favorites!
www.kriscarr.com

Ghost Mothers: Healing From the Pain of a Mother Who Wasn't Really There by Kathryn Rudlin, LCSW

Kathryn has a private practice in San Diego, CA specializing in providing support, education and healing to "ghost-mothered" women. (Sometimes physical health issues manifest when emotional issues are unresolved.) http://ghostmothers.com

Why Do I Still Have Thyroid Symptoms? When My Lab Tests are Normal by Datis Kharrazian, DHSc, DC, MS
This book is a revolutionary breakthrough in managing Hashimoto's and hypothyroidism. www.thyroid360.com

Why Isn't My Brain Working by Datis Kharrazian, DHSc, DC, MS
www.brainhealthbook.com

The Gluten Effect: How Innocent Wheat is Ruining your Health by Vikki and Richard Peterson, D.C., C.C.N. **www.healthnowmedical.com**

Not Just a Pretty Face: The Ugly Side of the Beauty Industry by Stacy Malkan
The book tells the inside story of the unprecedented research and advocacy efforts by the group of women who created the Campaign for Safe Cosmetics and built a national movement to shift the $50 billion beauty industry from harmful chemicals toward safer products.

(You can also find more information on how to give the beauty industry a makeover by visiting: www.safecosmetics.org)

The Whole Soy Story: the Dark Side of America's Favorite Health Food by Kaayla T. Daniel, Ph.D., C.C.N. www.kaayladaniel.com

Metamorphosis: Transforming your Body, Mind, and Life. by Dr. Charles Webb www.charleswebbdmp.com

5 Minute Stress Mastery Newsletter by Dr. Neil Neimark, M.D.
You will receive the latest practical, inspirational, and motivational breakthroughs for managing stress-related medical disorders and achieving greater health and healing for the mind, body and spirit. www.thebodysoulconnection.com

Grain Brain: The Surprising Truth about Wheat, Carbs, and Sugar–Your Brain's Silent Killers by Kristin Loberg and David Perlmutter www.drperlmutter.com

Recipe Books and Menus

There are many books, blogs, and websites to help you transition to an anti-inflammatory diet; here are my favorites.

Heart of Cooking by Sarah Schatz www.allergyfreemenuplanners.com
Allergy free and whole food menu planners for anyone on a limited diet.

Fresh from Elizabeth's Kitchen by Elizabeth Kaplan, founder of The Pure Pantry.
www.thepurepantry.com

Moms will appreciate the attention Elizabeth (mother of three kids) gives to kid-friendly recipes to include scrumptious dishes like spaghetti with turkey meatballs, veggie frittata, and lentil soup.

Autoimmune Paleo Cookbook: An Allergen-Free approach to Managing Chronic Illness by Mickey Trescott www.autoimmune-paleo.com
This is a book tailored to the anti-inflammatory diet.

Gluten-free Information

Dr. Thomas O'Bryan www.thedr.com **Celiac:** www.celiac.com
Dr. Thomas O'Bryan, DC, CCN, DACBM is an internationally recognized speaker and workshop leader specializing in Non-Celiac Gluten Sensitivity and Celiac Disease. I have the highest respect for his in-depth knowledge, passion, and extensive research as the "gluten guru".

Gluten Free Life by Linda Clark, M.A.,CNC www.ovitaminpro.com
Worthwhile tips on feeding your family, easy substitutions for thickeners, pastas, and snacks. This resource is full of yummy recipes, websites, cookbooks, and restaurants that offer gluten free menus.

Dealing with Environmental Toxins

EMF & RF Solutions: www.emfrf.com
Learn how to reduce electrosmog in your home.

Less EMF: www.lessemf.com
This site offers products to help shield yourself from harmful electrosmog.

Earthing: www.earthing.com
Earthing sells a variety of products, including the "universal mat" to help ground you to the earth.

PEMF (Pulsed Elektromagnetic Fields): www.pemf.com
This site provides information and education about anti-electrosmog technology and products. To inquire about your own anti-electrosmog in-home device or for sessions at my office, call us at 1-877-600-5222.

THYROSISTERS CHARITABLE CONTRIBUTIONS

Meet Mary and Bill, my folks. Their love story was about family, faith, education, health, and giving back to the community. Mary was a "health nut" during the time of Lindberg Nutrition and Adelle Davis. She strived to be vibrant and care for her three daughters. She taught the importance of love, hard work, and looking out for others. She was beautiful inside and out, and died of breast cancer before her time, at age 50.

Today the ThyroSisters "family" continues with Mom's tradition of excellence and humanitarianism. A portion of the profits of the sale of this book is donated to charitable causes.

You can view the causes that we contribute to at: www.ThyroSisters.com/Social-Responsibility.

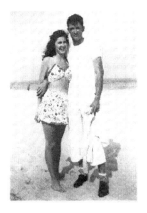

Mary and Bill

APPENDIX

Complete Blood Count (CBC)

- WBC
- RBC
- Hemoglobin
- Hematocrit
- Lymphocytes
- Monocytes
- MCH Mean
- MCHC Mean
- MCV Mean
- Neutrophils
- Platelets
- RDW

Thyroid Panel

- Total T-4 (Thyroxine)
- T-3 uptake
- Free-Thyroxine Index (FTI) T-7
- TSH
- TBG (Thyroid-binding globulin)
- TPO antibodies
- TGB antibodies
- FT3
- RT3

Lipid Profile

- Cholesterol, Total
- HDL
- LDL
- Cholesterol/HDL Ratio
- Triglycerides

Liver Profile

- Alanine aminotransferase (ALT or SGPT)
- Albumin
- Albumin/Globulin Ratio
- Alkaline Phosphatase
- Aspartate aminotransferase (AST or SGOT)
- Bilirubin, Total
- Globulin, Total
- Lactate Dehydrogenase (LDH)
- Protein, Total
- GGT

Kidney Panel

- Urea Nitrogen (BUN)
- Creatinine, Serum
- Uric Acid
- BUN/Creatinine

Minerals and Bone

- Iron, Total
- Calcium

- Phosphorus

Fluids and Electrolytes
- Chloride, Serum
- Potassium
- Sodium. Serum
- Carbon Dioxide

Diabetes
- Glucose

Thyroid Antibody Panel
- Anti-thyroglobulin
- Thyroid Peroxidase (TPO Ab)

NEUROLOGICAL TESTS

Blood pressure

Tissue oxygen saturation

Heart rate and rhythm

Saliva pH

Reflexes

Eye test

Cranial nerve tests

METABOLIC TESTS

Blood sugar levels

Adrenal function

Cortisol levels

Thyroid hormones

Cerebellar antibodies

Thyroid antibodies

Female hormone panel

Cerebellum tests

GI permeability test

Food allergies

Made in the USA
San Bernardino, CA
01 February 2020